EAT & THINK

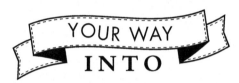

YOUR WAY

INTO

WEIGHT LOSS

Step By Step Action Guide & Journal

TAMI LINDAHL

Certified Biggest Loser Pro® & Weight Loss Specialist

www.TamiLindahl.com

Printed in the United States of America

Lindahl, Tami
Lose Weight, Transform Your Life: Eat and Think your way to Weight Loss – Step by step action guide and easy to follow plan for permanent weight loss.

by Tami Lindahl,
Certified Biggest Loser Pro® and Weight Loss Specialist
www.TamiLindahl.com

Contents

Note from the Author i

How to use this guide iii

Tools you will need to get started v

Goals, Commitments, and Motivation vi

Measurements: viii

Goal Setting ix

Commitment xii

Create your vision xiv

PART 1
Weight Loss Program

Introduction – Hormones and Weight Loss 1

Detoxifying Your Body 3

Fat Burning Foods 9

Healthy Mind, Healthy Body 21

Demystifying Label Reading 25

Call the Tooth Fairy 31

Good Carbs, Bad Carbs 33

The Good, The Bad and The Spicy 36

Portions 41

Plateaus and Road Blocks 45

Move Your Way Into Weight Loss 49

Stress and Weight Gain 53

Staying Motivated and Living Healthy 56

PART 2
Change Your Thinking, Transform Your Life

Step 1: Get the fire burning! 63

Step 2: Make a decision and move toward it! 65

Step 3: Think yourself thin!. 67

Step 4: Get out your MAP! 69

Step 5: Faith and affirmations. 71

Step 6: Getting real, and changing your limiting beliefs. 74

Step 7: Prayer, meditation and gratitude. 77

Step 8: Set yourself up for success! 79

Step 9: Surround yourself with winners! 81

Step 10: Persistence...Never give up! 83

PART 3
Journal

Daily Journals. 87

PART 4
Recipes

Breakfast Ziploc Omelets 173

Breakfast Yogurt. 174

Carrot Zucchini Pancakes 175

Quick and Easy Morning Oatmeal 176

Baked French Toast. 177

Eat the Good Fat First. 178

Spicy Almonds 179

Savory Olive Tapenade 180

Zesty Pesto Spread 181

Apple Cheddar Melts on Pita Toast 182

Ratatouille for Six. 183

Mini Greek Meatballs 184

Awesome Detox Soup 186

Lentil Soup 188

Spicy Yogurt Chicken 190

Pinto Bean Salad 192

Chicken with Apples and Leeks 194

Chicken and Basil 196

Easy veggie dip 198

Holiday Cranberry Sauce 199

Refreshing Mango Salsa 200

Salmon and Broccoli Stir Fry. 201

Sweet and Sour Chicken Recipe 202

Creamy Cauliflower Purée 205

Black Bean Brownies 207

Resources 209

Note from the Author

THANK YOU FOR choosing this book. It's the first step toward turning your body into a fat burning machine, having more energy and fitting into your skinny jeans again.

I have been in the fitness industry since 2001. My certifications include Certified Biggest Loser Pro ®, group exercise, personal training, kickboxing, youth and senior fitness, TRX, and lifestyle coaching, to name a few.

To date I've taught classes at the senior center, traditional gyms, women- only gyms, and in-home personal training. I've successfully run a "Fit Kids" program, been highlighted and published in several magazines and been a guest host on KHTS radio, including, the Fitness Hour with Ellen Como, the Senior Hour, and Beyond Harmony. I also sit on the board of the Health Care Committee through the SCV Chamber of Commerce.

In 2006 I opened my own gym called "Club 50 Fitness" that is, you guessed it; designed for men and women 50 and better. I've helped hundreds of people begin an exercise program, offered personal training to those who wanted more, and taught weekly weight loss classes. The more I learned about the weight loss program that I was offering at my gym, the more fascinated I became with learning about eating low glycemic foods. I eventually authored the book "How to Lose Weight without Being on a Diet, For Women"

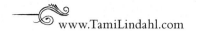

In July of 2011, I entered my and won my first NPC bikini competition in the Masters 45+ class. What an amazing and proud moment for me!

I now offer in-home personal training and coach people by phone. The phone coaching is a dynamic way to get the results you are looking for. The tools given in this guide are not just what to eat and how to move but they also give you what you need to stop sabotaging yourself so that you can have lasting results. Discover the fat burning foods so you can enjoy eating without guilt. Learn why diets don't work, and what does. With this step by step action guide and journal you will learn to enjoy living a healthy lifestyle and lose the weight you've always wanted in the process!

My next goal will be to open my ranch to you for total immersion to fitness, where you can come stay with me for a week or two and discover total fitness….

Tami Lindahl

www.FreeTrainerTips.com for health and fitness tips or to receive the newsletter.

For more info or training with Tami call 661-312-4239

How to use this guide

THIS BOOK IS designed to give you the information you need to understand what to eat and how to move but, it also gives insight to changing your life and keeping you inspired to not only reach your weight loss goals, but keep it off.

First, get all your measurements and pictures done, before you start any other part of the program. **Second**, when you sign your commitment and write out your motivation or vision, make a copy or two so you can see them both on a <u>daily</u> basis. *Take your time with these two exercises as they are going to keep you on track more than anything else.* **Third**, take this shopping and get everything you need right away!

As you begin to journal, write down what you ate and be sure to write the amount of what you ate. For example: protein- 3 oz. chicken breast, carb-½ cup white beans veggie- 1 cup steamed broccoli, fat- ¼ avocado; not just chicken with avocado, beans and broccoli. This will help you not only learn how to put your food in their right categories, but it will help your see where you need to add or subtract your foods.

It is very important to write down how you feel as well. Still hungry, tired, energized, craving sugar, depressed, feel good… Whatever it is, write it down so again, we can see a pattern on how certain foods affect you. At the bottom of

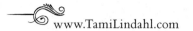

each page in the journal are famous quotes, health tips, or affirmations; use and enjoy them. The affirmations, or incantations, are something you can say over and over again to help you stay on track.

Tools you will need to get started

→ Bathroom scale that measures body fat

→ Tape measure

→ Kitchen scale for weighing food - nothing fancy

→ Be coachable, if you are open to the suggestions given in this program your journey will be more rewarding and successful. Things will feel and seem different (not normal), but remember *your* "normal" got you here.

→ Heart rate monitor

TIP: Always weigh and measure yourself at the same time of day, so your results will be most accurate. If you have someone else measure you, have the same person do it for the next measurement. Different people can equal different results and likely less accuracy.

Goals, Commitments, and Motivation

WRITING YOUR GOALS down actually signals your brain as to where you want to go. Your best chance of success is to be as clear as possible with what it is that you want. That goes with anything you want, not just weight loss. So how do you know what your goal should be? Here is your step by step plan to figure that out.

(a) Current weight

(b) Current % of body fat

(c) Current fat lbs.

(d) Lean body mass

(e) Fat % goal – between 20% to 30%; you decide

(f) Healthy amount of fat pounds

(g) Goal weight

1   (a) _____ x (b) _____ = (c) _____

2   (a) _____ – (c) _____ = (d) _____

3   (d) _____ x (e) _____%= (f) _____

4   (d) _____ + (f) _____ = (g) _____

5   (a) _____ – (g)= _____ fat lbs. to lose

Remember, you are losing fat not muscle, so the answer you came up with for fat lbs. to lose, is your target weight loss goal. So now you have both your goal weight and your weight loss goal. Keep them in mind, but don't let those big numbers scare you. You didn't get in your condition over-night nor will you rid the extra weight overnight. A realistic and healthy weight loss is no more than two pounds a week. If you are losing more than that, you may be losing muscle and you don't want that!! Also, fat takes up almost twice as much space as muscle so when you lose 10 lbs. of fat it will look like a loss of 20 lbs. when losing the *right* way.

Measurements:

USE THESE MEASURING tips as a guide to help you take your measurements, which should be recorded in your journal on Week 1, Day 1. Additional measurements should be taken during Weeks 3, 6, 9, and 12.

CHEST: Measure around the center of the breast (across the nipple) with bra on of course. If gravity has taken its course and the nipples are in... let's say... a different place, your arms can be up or down. Just make sure you measure the same way next time.

HIPS: Measure all the way around the largest part of your hips and butt, turning to your profile (side view) in the mirror to see where that is.

WAIST: Measure all the way around your waist, Use your navel as a point of reference.

BICEP: Measure from the top of the shoulder to the elbow. Take the mid-point as your location of measuring around the upper arm.

KNEE: Use a mirror and measure at the widest part of the knee

*Take a before picture now, front and profile.

Goal Setting

THE STARTING POINT of great success is when you sit down and decide exactly what you really want, in every area of your life. Continually set goals the rest of your life. Goals provide us with the challenges we need to keep our lives motivated. Being as specific as you can and creating real clarity for your brain will help you achieve what you want even faster!! Discovering what you really want, and stating what you really want, to achieve and being clear about it, in writing, your subconscious will find a way to get it!

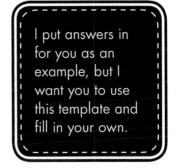

I put answers in for you as an example, but I want you to use this template and fill in your own.

What do I want to achieve?
(Long and short term goals)

I want to be at my optimum weight of 120lbs losing a total of 30 lbs(long term) I will lose 8 lbs this month (short term) I will lose 2lbs. this week (really short term)… set all 3!!… stay focused on the really short goal and your long term goal WILL come!!!

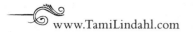
Why do I want to achieve this goal?

See attached worksheet… You must know your why!!! (See Motivation sheet on page xiv)

How will I achieve this goal? What is required to achieve this goal?

* *Go to the gym* - Go to the gym at least 3X a week - every Monday, Wednesday and Friday. I will spend 1 hour on cardio and half hour on strength training each session.
* *Eat healthier* - Eating foods that are low glycemic, and watch portions. Read all labels on foods before I buy them. Add healthy fat and avoid the "bad" fat
* *Regular detox* - Do the detox every 3 or 4 months
* *Get enough sleep* - Go to bed at 11pm every night and get up 6:30am
* *Do breathing exercise* - Spend 5 minutes on optimum breathing first thing when I get up
* *Get regular massage* - Go for massage every month (1st Friday of every month)
* *Play games* - Ride bikes with the kids, at Venice Beach every other Saturday
* *Take up Latin dancing… or country dancing … lol* ☺ - Sign-up for dance class once a week or go out dancing every Friday night.

When do I to achieve this goal?

**Put your new weekly goal where you can see it so you have that new number to look toward. Example: I want to achieve this goal by July 30th 2013 - 8 lbs. by May 30th – 2 lbs. by May 5th

What obstacles can I expect? (awareness is the key to growth)

- ✦ I am too tired when I get back from work to go to the gym.
- ✦ Pressure (or people) at work or home might affect my eating habits.
- ✦ I am too lazy sometimes to do any kind of exercise.
- ✦ I don't have time to eat healthy.

What are the solutions to the obstacles?

If you know how to combat the obstacle, the process becomes easier. You see it, you recognize it, and you know immediately what to do about it!

- ✦ Get up earlier and go to the gym before work, or put gym clothes in the car and go directly from work.
- ✦ Keep a diet journal to consciously be aware of what I am eating daily
- ✦ Get a gym or exercise buddy to motivate each other. Post on the forum, asking for help or offering some good ideas that work for you.
- ✦ Cut down unproductive time – spend only 1 hour per day for watching TV; buy pre cut frozen veggies so they are quick and easy to prepare.
- ✦ Keep only healthy food in the house. Pre cut frozen veggies are super easy...
- ✦ Tap into my subconscious mind and visualize that I am already healthy and fit before I go to bed at night... doing affirmations are great. Google low glycemic foods to keep your brain on track.
- ✦ Put a picture of a fit and trim self on my fridge ... or you doing activities that you can't currently do

Knowing your obstacles beforehand will help you know immediately when they surface and just what to do with them when they come so you don't get stuck! It's just a way of preparing yourself.

Commitment

IT IS IMPORTANT to have a commitment, even if it's to yourself. We make so many commitments to PTA, volunteering at the church, helping someone else with their kids, preparing food for your husband's office party, or maybe volunteering on a committee for a fundraiser. We are so good at helping other people; but it's time to commit to you. This is *your* time, time for you. If this is hard for you, remember, you can't take care of everyone else if you are not taking care of yourself. Think of it as being a role model for your family. If you show them you respect yourself, they will respect you for doing it. Begin by clearing out the junk food from your home (yes, the kids will live without potato chips in the house). Take a deep breath and go:

I _____

am making a commitment to myself and my fitness coach that:

+ I am making a commitment to change my life and my attitude.

+ I will follow instructions in this guide from my coach and be honest in my journal.

+ I will write in my journal daily.

+ I will finish the 12 week program.

+ I will not get discouraged if I have a bad day or do something I'm not supposed to do.

+ I will not compare myself for others.

+ I will not complain. I understand that everything in this program is to help me transform my life, my health and my body, for a life time!

+ I will exercise at *least* four days a week, or what ever my coach recommends for me.

_____

Print Name

_____

Signature

_____

Date

Create your vision

THIS IS PROBABLY one of the most important steps of all. I want you to now create the vision of what your life will look like a year from now if you lose the weight you want. What do your vacations look like? Are you finally comfortable in a bathing suit enjoying your family or significant other? Are you able to wear the clothes you want? What do they look like? Is your doctor able to take you off your blood pressure medication? How confident do you feel? Does that confidence show up in a more successful career? What do romantic situations feel like now that you lost the weight? Do you have your "sexy" back? Clarity is power so the more details the better!! If you are creating a vacation scenario, give details on where and what you are doing. Be sure to include feeling words so that you can really create an emotional connectedness to your story. The only way to predict the future is to create it, and this is how it starts…..

Create the life you want! (You may need a few sheets of paper for this one; go for it. This how you create your own future, the life you want, and it's really fun)

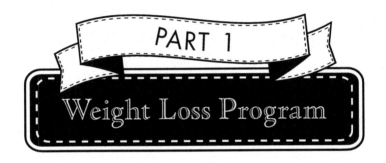

PART 1

Weight Loss Program

Introduction – Hormones and Weight Loss

AS WOMEN, WE deal with hormone issues throughout life beginning with puberty to our monthly visits from "Aunt Flo" to the mid life change. They affect us in so many ways, from cramping and bloating, fatigue, and irritability. Guys, you also have your issues with hormones as well. They have an effect on our weight. Insulin, thyroid and cortisol all regulate our body's ability to go into fat storage or fat burning modes. Many of our hormones are not under our control but many of them are.

When we have high levels of the hormone insulin it signals our body to store fat. In addition if we continue to keep our insulin levels up by eating high glycemic foods we are on a fast track to insulin resistance and possible diabetes type II. I'll be talking about how to keep the levels steady.

Our thyroid regulates our metabolism, which is our body's ability to efficiently burn calories. A low thyroid level will slow the thyroids function and tell the body to burn calories at a slower rate.

Cortisol is our "belly fat" hormone. This one is controlled by keeping our stress levels in check. Increased levels

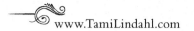

of cortisol tell the body to store fat around the mid section and also keep us from getting a decent night's sleep. Lack of sleep can also stress us out and lead to weight gain, so it's a vicious cycle.

Weigh loss is not about going on a diet and hoping for the best. It's about learning to eat and exercise in a way that turns your body into a fat burning machine. The goal is to create a healthy mindset so you can keep it off, which will be addressed in part 2 of this guide.

This step by step action guide is intended to provide you with tips to keep your body in a fat burning mode. It is not a "diet," but a lifestyle that you can live with long term. Simple choices that you make daily and consistently will have your metabolism revved up and burning fat so you never have to diet again!

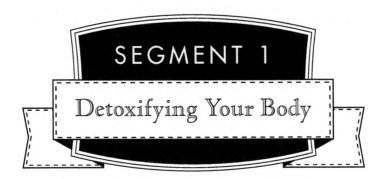

SEGMENT 1

Detoxifying Your Body

A S WE GO through life, we breathe in smog, eat processed foods, and consume sugars, sugar substitutes, alcohol, fats, chemicals, and other toxins. These get trapped in
our bodies and in our fat cells. These unhealthy consump-
tions can cause poor nutrient absorption, and puts a lot of
stress on the liver and digestive tract. With poor nutrient absorption, your body thinks it's starving and craves more food
which leads to over eating. Think of detoxing as re-booting
your metabolism. The liver has two jobs; one is to detoxify
the body and the other is to metabolize fat. Once your system is "clean" the fat metabolizing efforts of your liver will
function so much better.

During this first week you will be eliminating the toxins
from your diet and ultimately your body. This is the toughest
week of the entire program but probably the most important
to get you set up for success. Without the "junk" in your
system the cravings for sugars, carbs, or processed food will
subside. So the better you stick with this the easier the next
11 weeks will be! Toxins are stored in your fat cells, so you
will see an immediate drop in weight this week.

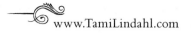

Here are your steps:

1 Start your day with a cup of hot water with the juice of half a lemon.

2 Eat only cleansing foods which are mostly vegetables (eat as much as you want), and some fruit (limit your fruit to three servings a day). This is not about going hungry, so eat! You can add lean chicken, fish or lean sources of protein. Also, you can enjoy the detox soup that is found in the "Recipes" section of this book.

3 Avoid salt, oils, butter, bread, cereal, rice, beans, pasta, sugar, sugar substitutes, caffeine, alcohol, dairy, and red meat.

4 Be prepared! Have your soup or your veggies with you so you don't end up at the fast food place.

5 Drink lots of water! Figure one-half an ounce per pound of body weight. So if you're 150lbs. you want to be sure you drink at least 75 oz per day!

6 Get lots of rest this week. The detoxification process may leave you tired and sluggish. Don't worry; that's normal.

7 Don't start (or continue) your exercise program this week. Instead get a massage or pamper yourself. This is a tough week, so be kind to yourself. If you must do something, try some simple stretches, gentle yoga, or go for a walk.

8 Detox your kitchen and get rid of any and all junk food. If you can't bring yourself to throw it away, make it really hard to reach... so you don't "accidentally" eat it.

You have not failed; your diets have failed you!

Have you yo-yo dieted only to gain more weight back than you started with? Most well known diets enable people to lose weight, but why do they always gain the weight back? The good news is that you have not failed; your diets have. They cause you to lose muscle, which is the *last* thing you want to lose. Muscle is what helps your body efficiently burn calories. Let's talk about some of them...

Let's start with the **low calorie** diet. Severely restricting your calories puts your body in "starvation mode." Your body doesn't know that there is a fridge full of food so your brain will tell your thyroid to slow down and hang on to body fat, thereby burning muscle. You have now just slowed your metabolism by 10% to 15%. The last thing you want to do is to burn muscle. The more efficient your metabolism is, the better your body burns calories. So I always say "muscle dictates metabolism."

How about the **"low carb"** diet? People have been losing weight on this one for a while now. This one has you eating lots of protein but omitting whole grains, fruit and vegetables. This is a very dangerous and unhealthy way to eat and again, will create muscle loss instead of fat. What do you think your cholesterol will look like if you are eating high fat foods and getting no fiber? Your brain needs glucose (sugar) to function so if you aren't eating your healthy carbs your body will make it any way.

Then there are the **meal replacement** diets. "Have a shake for breakfast, a shake for lunch and then have a sensible dinner". First of all, if we had that much control to not "eat"

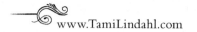
anything until our sensible dinner we wouldn't be in this mess in the first place. Again this diet will only have you losing muscle and not body fat. Say it with me "muscle dictates metabolism." These shakes are usually high in sugar and how long can anyone stick with it? Studies have shown that 95% of people on this diet will gain the weight back the first year and 97% will gain it back by the second year. It is just a quick fix and that won't last long term.

I'm sure if you're reading this, chances are you have tried some of the other well known diets. The main thing these diets have in common is that they are *diets* and they **don't** have you losing fat, just muscle. You know the saying "muscle dictates metabolism!" This is why diets don't work. So, it's really about getting in good habits and breaking old ones. This program is the perfect start for that!

Here is your shopping list:

Produce: (Go all organic)

- ✦ Asparagus
- ✦ Bell peppers (red is the most nutritious)
- ✦ Broccoli
- ✦ Cauliflower
- ✦ Cabbage (red or green or both)
- ✦ Carrots
- ✦ Garlic, fresh
- ✦ Green beans
- ✦ Lemons
- ✦ Lettuce (romaine, spring mix, mixed greens. Just not iceberg)
- ✦ Onion, leeks and scallions
- ✦ Radishes
- ✦ Snap or snow peas
- ✦ Spinach
- ✦ Tomatoes
- ✦ Zucchini

Pretty much any veggies you like will work, especially this week

Carbs: (Go organic)

- ✦ Fruit : Apples, berries, oranges, lemons, limes, grapefruit, peaches, plums etc.
- ✦ Yams or sweet potatoes
- ✦ Peas
- ✦ Winter squash like acorn, butternut or spaghetti squash

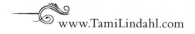

Protein: (Go organic, or free range)

+ Chicken breast or ground chicken breast
+ Turkey or ground turkey breast
+ Eggs
+ Fish (swai, or tilapia. You can also include shrimp or other seafood.)
+ Edamame

This is for this week only. You will be adding more carbs next week. Try to get all organic when possible, remember you are ridding your body of toxins and non-organic foods are full of pesticides, hormones and other chemicals!!

Fat:

+ Raw nuts, ground flax seed
+ Olive & coconut oil
+ Avocado

Miscellaneous:

+ SweetLeaf ® Stevia
+ Detox tea
+ Vinegar (I like balsamic, but you choose)

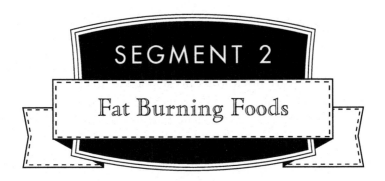

SEGMENT 2

Fat Burning Foods

Choosing Low Glycemic foods

O K, LET'S TALK about how you *will* be eating. I've talked about the different diets and why they don't work, so what I want to share with you is more of a lifestyle, not a diet. When I first started teaching this low glycemic program in my fitness center, I lost 12 lbs. almost through osmosis. Just learning how to make better choices and making subtle changes to my diet, I couldn't help but lose a few pounds – without feeling deprived at all!

You'll be choosing your foods based on the glycemic impact they have on your body. We're not counting calories (although eating too much of anything causes weight gain). When you eat anything that will quickly spike your blood sugar levels, your body automatically goes into a "fat storage mode." Eating high glycemic foods will raise your insulin levels, which signals the body to store fat. Eating foods that are low glycemic will help your body stay in a "fat burning" mode.

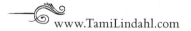

Food list

Here is a short list of foods that are lower glycemic and fat burning foods. You will choose one <u>protein</u>, one <u>fat</u> and one <u>carb</u>. <u>Veggies</u> are an "all you can eat" food so fill up on them. Understanding how to divide your food into these four categories will help you understand how to put your meals together, be healthy and NOT be on a diet!

Veggies:

✦ Alfalfa sprouts, Chard, Lettuce- (any) Artichokes, Collard greens, Mushrooms

✦ Asparagus, Cucumber, Okra , Bean/broccoli sprouts, Eggplant, Olives

✦ Bell peppers, Endive, Onions, Broccoli Green beans, Snow peas, Brussels sprouts

✦ Hot peppers, Spinach, Cabbage (red or green), Jicama, String beans

✦ Cauliflower, Kale, Tomatoes, Celery, Leeks, Zucchini

✦ ★Winter Squash (butternut, spaghetti & acorn)

✦ ★Sweet potatoes/ Yams

✦ ★Peas

★These are starches, and fall into the "carb" category, so choose these instead of rice or potato. Only fill one-fourth of your plate with these, or **"one serving"** per meal.

Most veggies are OK, just avoid, parsnips, corn, white and brown potatoes, and turnips as they are medium to high glycemic.

Carbs:

On these you will want to stick to one serving per meal. Unlike most of the veggies this is not an "all you can eat" type of food. Typically one-half cup is a serving, or one-fourth of your plate. Eat your carbs in the morning, think of them as your energy for the day. You don't need "energy" at the end of the day, so skipping a carb at dinner is recommended.

Fruit:

A serving is one medium fruit unless otherwise noted. Consider fruit as a carb.

Enjoy:

→ Apples, four medium Apricots, Grapefruit, Mandarin Oranges, ¾ of a cup of Grapes, Nectarines, Banana (green), one-sixteenth of a Honeydew, Med Oranges, ¾ of a cup of Berries (all kinds)

→ Kiwi, Peaches, four Kumquats, Pears, twelve Cherries, Lemons, Persimmons, Limes, half of a medium Papaya, 2 Figs (fresh), seven Lychees

→ Plums, Pomegranates

Avoid: Raisins, ripe bananas, water melon.

→ Eat your fruit rather than drink it. Sure, you get all the vitamins but all the fiber is removed which makes it high glycemic.

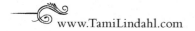
Beans:

One serving is ½ cup

→ *Enjoy:* Red, black, garbanzo (chick peas), lima beans, mung, fava, kidney, navy, pinto, soy beans, green and black eyed peas and lentils and split peas.

→ *Avoid:* Refried beans, pork and beans, or baked beans with sugar added.

Grains:

One serving is ½ cup

→ *Enjoy:* Barley, bran (oat or rice wheat), breads that are high fiber, low carb, stone ground or sprouted. Bulgur wheat, pasta that is high fiber /protein (cooked aldente'), steamed brown rice.

→ *Occasionally:* Buckwheat and other whole grain noodles, cornmeal, and couscous.

→ *Avoid:* White or wheat flour, most breads, boiled rice (brown or white) millet, bagels, cookies, donuts, cake, and other dessert like or sugary foods.

Cereals:

→ *Enjoy:* (Low carb, high protein), rolled oats (oatmeal), All bran, Bran buds, cream of wheat, Complete Bran Flakes, muesli or granola with no sugar added.

→ *Avoid:* Cheerios, Corn flakes, Rice Krispies, anything processed, added sugar, or instant.

→ I would also recommend including a lean protein if you are having this for breakfast. It will keep you fuller much longer. Eating carbs for breakfast, even the good ones, can have you feeling hungry long before lunch.

Protein:

Typically four to six ounces is one serving, which should be about 20 grams of protein.

→ *Enjoy:* Chicken, fish, beef, veal, turkey, tofu, seafood, Canadian bacon, eggs or egg whites, liquid egg substitutes.

→ *Avoid:* Sausage, bacon, chicken skin, or any type or meat with a lot of visible fat

Dairy and substitutes:

→ *Enjoy:* Nonfat cheese, cottage cheese, almond milk (watch the sugar) oat milk, low or non fat milk, plain yogurt with no sugar added. Check your serving size.

→ *Avoid:* Yogurts with fruit and sugar/ sugar substitutes. I simply add my own fruit, vanilla extract, and a little agave syrup, or Stevia to plain yogurt so I know what I'm getting, plus it tastes good.

Fats:

Choose just one serving per meal

→ *Go for:* Coconut oil, olive oil, flaxseed oil, walnut oil, grape seed oil, nuts (all), avocado, ground flax or hemp seed, and salmon.

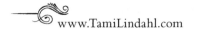

✦   *Avoid:* dairy fat like cheese, vegetable oil, margarine (most), partially hydrogenated, or hydrogenated oils.

All fats are higher in calories than protein or carbs so be sure to measure what a serving is before you douse your food with it.

★Butter is in its own class. It's saturated, but it is a natural fat, so use it sparingly. I will say that I do prefer it to most margarines.

Condiments:

✦   *Enjoy:* Vinegar, lemon juice, mustard, horseradish, salsa, hot sauce, agave syrup.

✦   *Avoid:* Ketchup, sauces like teriyaki & BBQ, mayonnaise, pancake syrup.

Breakfast ideas:

EXAMPLE 1:   Egg white omelet★ (2 to 5 egg whites), with veggies, at least ½ cup or more, such as: broccoli, carrots, spinach, mushrooms, onion, tomatoes, peppers, whatever veggies you like, and as much as you like.

★Egg whites have about 20 calories, zero fat and 4 grams of protein. While the whole egg contains as much as 100 calories, 5 grams of fat (2 grams Saturated) and 6 grams protein. As you can see your real protein source is the egg whites and your fat and calories come from the yolk, so go white as much as you can. If you add one whole egg count that yolk as your one serving of fat.

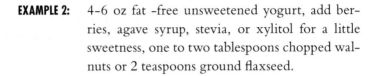

EXAMPLE 2: 4-6 oz fat -free unsweetened yogurt, add berries, agave syrup, stevia, or xylitol for a little sweetness, one to two tablespoons chopped walnuts or 2 teaspoons ground flaxseed.

★see recipes for yogurts ideas.

EXAMPLE 3: 4-6 oz. non-fat cottage cheese, sprinkled with ground flaxseed. 2-3 cups veggies, either mixed in or on the side.

EXAMPLE 4: Oatmeal with egg whites and sliced almonds (adding a whole egg includes your fat requirement so skip the nuts), cinnamon, vanilla or almond extract, and a little stevia

Lunch/ dinner ideas:

Include a lean protein, as many veggies as you like, one low GI carb, and one fat.

EXAMPLE 1: 4-6 oz. skinless chicken breast, steamed asparagus with mushrooms and almonds, and ½ cup lentils

EXAMPLE 2: Big salad with lots of veggies, ½ cup garbanzo beans and 4-6 oz. grilled salmon, or lean beef, or chicken. Top with a tablespoon of olive oil and vinegar.

EXAMPLE 3: Broiled or grilled shrimp or scallops, a side salad and steamed broccoli and cauliflower and ½ baked yam. (or one small yam) lightly drizzled with coconut oil

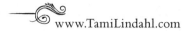

Snacks:

Combine a carb and fat, a fat and protein, or protein and carb. Just don't have a carb by itself.

EXAMPLE 1:   Raw or grilled mixed veggies, with a drizzle of olive oil

EXAMPLE 2:   Fruit or veggies with 1-2 oz. non fat cottage cheese

EXAMPLE 3:   Hummus and veggies

EXAMPLE 4:   Apple or celery with peanut butter

EXAMPLE 5:   1 serving of dark chocolate with strawberries

Having a carb by itself will raise your blood sugars and have you hungrier by the next meal unless you add a fat or protein! You can always add veggies to any of your snacks or meals; did I mention they are on the "all you can eat" list? ☺

Here is your new shopping list:

(after your 1 week detox)

Produce: Go all organic, when you can ….

+ Broccoli
+ Cauliflower
+ Cabbage red or green or both!
+ Carrots
+ Garlic, fresh
+ Green beans
+ Lettuce like romaine, spring mix, mixed greens. Just not iceberg
+ Onion, or leeks and scallions
+ Peppers, all, like bell, padilla, or jalapeño
+ Radishes
+ Spinach
+ Tomatoes
+ Zucchini

Carbs:

+ Fruit: apples, oranges, berries, plums, peaches, lemons, apricots, cherries etc.
+ Yams or sweet potatoes
+ Winter squash like acorn, butternut or spaghetti squash
+ Beans (canned is ok, just no sugar added) like garbanzo, black, navy or white or kidney
+ Brown rice, Quinoa
+ Peas
+ Oatmeal

Protein:

+ Chicken breast, or ground chicken breast
+ Turkey or ground turkey breast
+ Eggs
+ Fish, such as swai, or tilapia. You can also include shrimp or other seafood.
+ Salmon (which is also a fat as well as a protein)
+ Edamame or tofu
+ Non fat Greek yogurt NO sugar added, or non fat cottage cheese
+ Protein powder, or a protein shake (I like Blue Bonnet ®)

Fat:

+ Olive & coconut oil
+ Avocados
+ Dark chocolate
+ Ground flax or hemp seeds
+ Nuts, raw

Condiments:

+ SweetLeaf® Stevia, packets or flavored drops
+ Mustard, salsa, horseradish
+ Spices: ginger, cumin, curry, chili powder, cinnamon
+ Extracts, like vanilla or maple
+ Vinegar (no sugar added)

Here is your new shopping list after week 6:

Everything on the other list only now you can add:

Carbs:

Barley
Low glycemic bread, like Ezekiel
100% whole grain tortilla
Low glycemic pasta (or 100% whole grain, high fiber)

★★Going gluten free the 1st six weeks is helpful in knowing whether you are gluten intolerant or not.

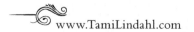

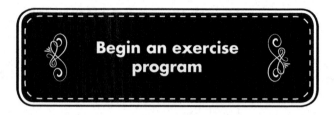

Begin an exercise program

If you are new to exercise, I highly recommend hiring a trainer. You don't want to start out with bad habits and end up hurting yourself. At a minimum, join a gym that offers classes so you can talk to the instructor and let her know you are new and advise her of any limitations you may have. I know this may seem intimidating, but swallow your pride and ask as many questions as you can. Believe me, as an instructor myself, I really appreciated people coming to me with their questions or concerns, and frankly, I had more respect for them.

Also be sure to include both cardio and resistance type exercise. Cardio alone will not do the trick. Remember earlier, we talked about muscle dictating metabolism, so it's very important that we do what it takes to get those lean muscles!

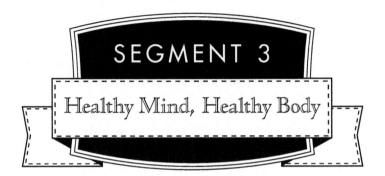

SEGMENT 3

Healthy Mind, Healthy Body

YOU NEED TO set a goal, but first you need to realize where you are, and where you want to go. Is your goal to be thin, the end all, be all, and your deepest desire, or is your goal to maximize your health and improve quality of life?

Ask yourself:

1   Is my goal just to be thin?

2   Is my goal realistic?

3   What is my attitude about fat and weight loss?

4   What am I (if anything) willing to change about my behaviors to achieve these goals?

Your goals should be realistic. For example if you are losing more than two pounds a week you will not have long term success. One to two pounds is plenty. Remember if you lose too fast, you will be losing muscle which will come back to "bite" you later.

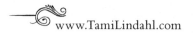

Making new habits:

I will _____ **daily** to achieve my goal. Example: (scheduling exercise, journaling, pack my lunch for work, keep my workout clothes in my car, be prepared with healthy choices, etc.)

I will _____ **weekly** to achieve my goals. Example: (plan meals and your shopping trip with a list, check in with your coach, etc.)

I will _____ **monthly** to achieve my goals. Example: (Re-evaluate your exercise plan and possibly increasing intensity, mode or duration, weigh and measure myself, etc.)

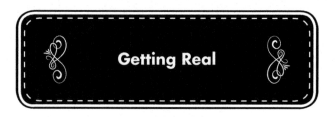

1 **Do you believe that once you reach a certain weight or size you will be happy?** The old saying goes "wherever you go there you are." So if you are waiting to lose the weight to be happy, I can tell you now, you will be disappointed. So what do you do? First, go easy on yourself. Take joy in the two pounds lost or the looseness in your pants. Acknowledge yourself for showing up to your workout when you didn't "feel like it," take note of how good you feel about yourself when you say "no thank you" to something you may

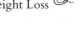

have automatically said yes to only to later feel that tremendous guilt. This is about progress, NOT perfection!!

2 **Do you use excuses for making bad food choices or not to exercise?** Do you find yourself saying "I don't have time to exercise," "the rest of my family would never eat that," I don't like to get sweaty" or "I'll start Monday?" This is what I call limiting beliefs. If you believe them to be true, then they are. *So here is your assignment*: write down all your limiting beliefs, and then write the solution. If you believe you don't have time then write a way to make time, etc. I believe in you and I believe this will empower you tremendously.

3 **Are you afraid of disappointing others?** The truth is, when you begin to make these changes, some will be very supportive and some won't be so thrilled, however, that is their issue, not yours. You may experience feelings of guilt, or fear of disapproval, but taking care of yourself is not just your right, it's your responsibility.

4 **Do you find yourself procrastinating?** If your answer is yes, then this is just fear. Fear of failure, fear of success, fear of what people will think of you when you do lose the weight, fear of doing it wrong or not being "perfect" in your efforts... you get the picture. I'm looking for progress, not perfection. So, if you just move forward and do what is suggested to the best of your ability, you'll do just fine. I could ask what will happen if you do nothing? What if you don't do what's asked of you in this program? Not only will you keep the weight on, but chances are you'll continue to gain more... so, ready or not, go ahead and jump in.

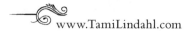

5 **Beware of family and friends**. You may here things such as:

- "Oh, come on, a little won't hurt you."
- "I made this just for you."
- "It's my birthday, just have a little."
- "Let's go to happy hour or out for a few drinks."
- "Skipping exercise just this once won't make a difference."
- And my personal favorite "You're looking too thin". I bet the person who says that is bigger than you...

The reactions of people closest to you will vary, but I wanted to give you a few ideas on what sabotage looks like. Most of the time it will come from the people who also have issues with their weight and by you doing something positive for yourself, they are forced to look in the mirror. To them, it feels like you are making them look bad and that's why they do it. My advice here is to get your family, office workers or whoever you are in close contact with and tell them exactly what you are doing. Go ahead and come right out and ask for their support. If you ask them, they are most likely to want to help you. Turn it around; if someone asks you for help, especially as a woman, don't you want to go out of your way to help them?

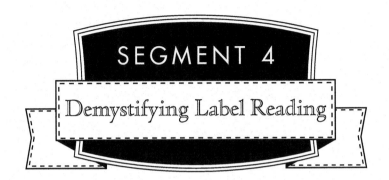

SEGMENT 4

Demystifying Label Reading

Reading makes you skinny...

I KNOW, I KNOW... who has time to read labels? With a full time job, kids, and household chores there is little time to stop and read labels. All I can say (like with exercise) is take the time. Once you start to read labels you will be shocked at what's actually in your food. There are hidden sugars and fats everywhere! Take cereal for example. Which is your best choice, Smart Start or Lucky Charms? The answer is neither! When you look on the label of Smart Start you'll find it has more sugar than Lucky Charms! Yikes! Don't even get me started on the Lucky Charms. Who's idea was it to give children marshmallows for breakfast anyway? Be sure to scan the whole label. You may see something labeled low fat, but after further inspection you see it's high in sugar and calories. Just because something is labeled a "diet food" that doesn't mean it's good for you or even going to help you lose weight.

Label reading tips:

✦ Check your serving size. Sometimes what appears to be a single serving is two or more which will double (or more) the fat, sugars and calories.

+ No more than 120 carbs (aim for 30 per meal) a day, and make sure they are the healthy kind; beans, yams, barley, high protein/fiber pasta, oatmeal, legumes, 100% whole grain or flourless bread. You can definitely go for less to speed up your weight loss, just don't cut them all out. No more than 33% of your daily intake from fat, but make it the good kind. Olive or coconut oil, nuts, avocados, fish oil or flaxseeds.

+ Look for foods with no trans fat, and little to no saturated fat, consume no more than 20 grams of saturated fat per day. One of the biggest sources of saturated fat is from animals, from the fat in the meat to the fat in butter or other dairy products. Go for non-fat versions of dairy products. We'll add the "good fat" into your diet, we just don't want too much of the saturated kind.

+ When deciding which products have to much fat, look for the DV% (Daily Value). It should say no more than 10% (saturated) or that 30% of the calories are from fat, unless you are looking at the label on nuts or olive oils or any of your omega three's. Those are your good fats and they promote weight loss when you make it the first part of your meal and in the right portions.

+ Fiber is your friend! For women you need about 25 grams a day and men need about 35grams. When eating something with lots of fiber, not only will it keep you full, but, it lowers the glycemic impact of your food. So for breads, pastas or cereals go for the ones with the highest fiber, and lowest sugar content.

+ Check the sugar content. It's everywhere. Check for it on your can of beans, yogurt, breads, tortillas, soups, salad dressings, and other marinades or sauces. If the label says it has 12 grams of sugar then you divide by four, to get the amount of teaspoons of sugar; this product would have three teaspoons of sugar (per serving)… how many servings are you eating?

Label reading lingo

✦   Low calorie = One-third the calories of the original version or similar product

✦   Lite =One-third the calories or half the fat of the original or similar product

✦   Organic= Simply stated, organic produce and other ingredients are grown without the use of pesticides, synthetic fertilizers, sewage sludge, genetically modified organisms, or ionizing radiation. Animals that produce meat, poultry, eggs, and dairy products do not take antibiotics or growth hormones.

The USDA National Organic Program (NOP) defines organic as follows:

Organic food is produced by farmers who emphasize the use of renewable resources and the conservation of soil and water to enhance environmental quality for future generations. Organic meat, poultry, eggs, and dairy products come from animals that are given no antibiotics or growth hormones. Organic food is produced without using most conventional pesticides; fertilizers made with synthetic ingredients or sewage sludge; bioengineering; or ionizing radiation. Before a product can be labeled "organic,"

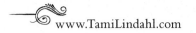

a government-approved certifier inspects the farm where the food is grown to make sure the farmer is following all the rules necessary to meet USDA organic standards. Companies that handle or process organic food before it gets to your local supermarket or restaurant must be certified, too.

✦ High fiber = Five grams or more per serving

✦ No preservatives added = Does not contain added chemicals. It may contain natural preservatives like sodium.

Buzz words...

When you look at the nutritional information on your labels, you will see that your product has fat, or sugars or carbs. Not all fats sugars and carbs are bad... It's their source we are most concerned with. The best way to know what you're getting is to start by reading your ingredient list. As we learn to read labels we look for "buzz words" that we either like or don't like to see on our ingredient list. Here are a few:

Avoid:

High glycemic

✦ Instant

✦ Enriched flour

✦ White flour

✦ Bleached flour

✦ Wheat flour

✦ Malodexrtins

✦ Modified food starch

Go for:

Low glycemic

✦ Original (oatmeal)

✦ Stone ground

✦ 100% Whole grain

✦ Buckwheat, whole rye

✦ Sprouted

✦ Flourless

✦ Pickled or vinegar

Avoid:

Sugars

+ High fructose corn syrup
+ Sugar, honey
+ Corn syrup/ solids
+ Brown sugar
+ Evaporated cane syrup
+ Brown rice syrup
+ Organic cane juice

Sweeteners

+ Aspartame

+ Saccharine

Fats

+ Trans fat
+ Canola oil

+ Partially hydrogenated
+ Hydrogenated
+ Shortening
+ Palm kernel oil
+ Butter

Go for:

Sugars

+ Fruit, like raisins

+ Agave

Sweeteners

+ Sucralose in moderation, it's a chemical
+ Stevia, or reb A
+ Xylitol, or other sugar alcohols

Fats

+ Coconut milk
+ Flaxseed, or hempseeds ground
+ Coconut or olive oil
+ Nuts (any)
+ Walnut oil
+ Palm fruit oil
+ Sunflower oil
+ Avocado

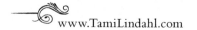

So when you see on your ingredient list on your bread labels "stone ground", or "sprouted" you will know that's probably a good choice. But when you see "enriched" or "wheat flour" you will know it's a high glycemic food and that it will put your body in fat storage!

If you see your product has a lot of fat but all you see on the top of the ingredient list is nuts, you know that it may very well be a good choice. Sometimes you will see things from both columns and you will have to make a choice from there, just look at the ingredient list order.

Anything on your ingredient list is put in the order of the most to the least. So if high fructose corn syrup is near the top of the ingredient list, then it has more than we want (we don't really want any). However, if it's at the bottom of the ingredient list, then it's something we may consider eating. Copy this list and bring it on your next shopping trip. You may be surprised what's in your food!

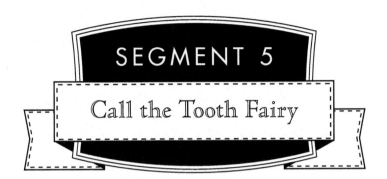

SEGMENT 5

Call the Tooth Fairy

ARE YOU A sugar addict? Do you feel like you just need to eat something sweet after almost every meal? Well, most of us have gone through this in our dieting journey. Sugar or sweet is an addition. The less sweet or sugar you have, the less you'll crave. This is one of the main reasons the detox is so important. If you go without sugar (and sugar substitutes) for the week, your craving will subside. After six weeks, a fresh apple or strawberries will taste as sweet as candy, and the candy won't taste as good. If you find you are still craving sugars, extend or do another detoxify. Don't worry, this does get easier.

Sugars are everywhere and we need to be aware of just how much sugar we're taking in every day. How much soda are you drinking every day? Are you addicted to carbs like breads, potatoes and pasta? These turn to sugar immediately in your body, and you guessed it, puts you in fat storage. More importantly, eventually you will become insulin resistant and that's a dangerous road which can lead to diabetes. Diet sodas are no better! Studies have shown people who drink diet sodas are actually fatter than those who didn't. One study gave one group of rat's water, one group soda, and the other group diet soda. They gave all three groups the equivalent of chocolate cake. The rats that just had water ate some and stopped, the other two groups ate all the cake until it was gone! The sweet taste had become an addiction.

As I mentioned last week, reading labels is key. Not just how many grams per serving but, where on the ingredients list is the sugar source? If it's high on the list, it's mostly sugar. The sources could be: sugar, brown sugar, high fructose corn syrup, brown rice syrup, corn syrup, honey etc. Sugar substitutes should be avoided as much as possible now, too. The worst offenders are aspartame or saccharine. If you must have it, go for stevia, sucralose, or xylitol. My personal favorite sweetener is stevia, and agave syrup. Agave syrup is very similar to honey but because it doesn't spike your blood sugar levels, it is low glycemic. It is not calorie free, so use it sparingly.

My most important message to you in this segment is that I'd really like to see you cut out as many sweets (calorie free or otherwise) as possible, so that you don't have that sugar tooth any more. This will make a huge difference in your weight loss success!

OK, with that said, you are not doomed to never have a bit of birthday cake now again. I just want you to be able to say to yourself "I don't eat sweets," and feel good about it.

If your are headed to a party or event that will be offering sweets, have a little if you must, then pop some gum in your mouth to make it less tempting to eat more.

Once you begin your "mental conditioning" you won't want the sweets nearly as much, so you can call the tooth fairy because you <u>will</u> lose that sugar tooth. I will go more into that in part 2 of the book but basically what you believe will determine your behavior, which will of course, determine your results.

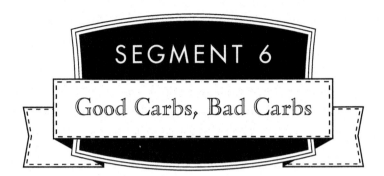

SEGMENT 6

Good Carbs, Bad Carbs

THE QUESTION MOST often asked is "how many carbs should I eat at one sitting?" The answer is, it depends. If you are moderately active, then you'll want about 30-50 grams per meal and 30 grams per snack. For weight loss purposes I would recommend you not exceed 30 grams per meal and 10-15 per snack, staying within 120 per day. These numbers are just FYI... This program is designed to be as easy to follow as possible, so there is no need to be counting anything. If you make it a basic rule to have one serving of good carb per meal you should be fine. The most important part of this equation is to choose the right carbs and avoid the bad ones. You'll find your list and servings sizes in segment two.

You need your carbs, but we just want to be sure they are the right ones. And really if you focus on eating lots of veggies and fruit you won't need these other carbs. Once you get to week six, you can now include some of the other carbs we left out in week two. You can now add in, whole grain tortillas or breads, steamed brown rice, and whole wheat pasta and barley. These all are full of gluten so you may choose to stay off them completely if being off them felt better. Always look for the highest fiber version of these pastas, breads and tortillas. Check your buzz word list for your clues as to what

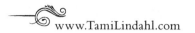

your best choices of carb are, such as sprouted, flourless, stone ground, low glycemic, etc.

Another key tip here is to eat your carbs toward the end of the meal, or at least don't start with it. When you are hungry and your stomach is empty your blood sugars are low. If you eat a high glycemic food item first, it will immediately spike your insulin levels and put your body in a fat storing zone. Everything you eat from here on out will be stored as fat. Your best bet is to start your meals with a healthy fat like avocado, nuts, olive oils, or flaxseed. If you are going to have toast (whole grain high fiber or low glycemic is best of course) for breakfast, sprinkling some ground flaxseed or spreading almond butter or avocado on it changes its glycemic impact and keeps you out of the fat storage zone. Do not just have a carb alone for breakfast; be sure to include a protein to keep you satisfied till lunch. As with all your meals, keep them balanced: one protein, one carb, one healthy fat, and all the veggies you can eat! If you skip a carb in the evening, that's fine. Just don't skip them altogether.

When you are journaling or putting your meals together, you are simply taking one item from each of the categories. Even if you are not choosing something from the "enjoy " list, (life happens, right?) at least if you stick to **ONE serving** of the "bad" carbs, you won't stray too far off track. Obviously, these should be avoided, but if you have them, know your category and your serving size and stick to one serving.

This is a list of some common carbs that may find their way onto your plate. At least once you know their category it will help you make your best choices...

Consider these carbs:

- ✦ Bread ,1 slice, 1 roll, any kind, good or bad
- ✦ Couscous ½ cup
- ✦ ★Corn or potato chips, about 15 chips
- ✦ Corn -½ cup
- ✦ Crackers of any kind –check package for serving size
- ✦ Hamburger or hotdog buns – ½ the bun
- ✦ Popcorn (★with butter)- 3 cups popped
- ✦ Pizza (dough) 1 slice ★with cheese
- ✦ Potatoes; whole, mashed or ★fried – 1 potato or ½ cup mashed
- ✦ Refried , or baked beans ½ cup
- ✦ Rice or pasta of any kind ½ cup
- ✦ Tortilla or ★tortilla shell or chips

★Consider these a fat as well. So if you are at the Mexican restaurant, and you have the chips and salsa, for example, you have filled your carb and fat categories so the rest of your meal should be only be protein and veggies. I would prefer you get your fat from the guacamole, and your carb from the whole beans, (which is the BEST choice) but life is about choice so if you have the chips you'll just skip the guacamole and beans… just this once right? ☺

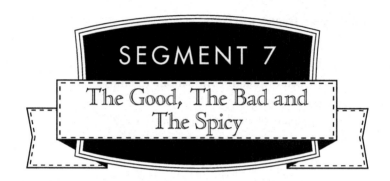

SEGMENT 7

The Good, The Bad and The Spicy

Spice up your life!

KEEPING YOUR FAT intake in check doesn't mean giving up on flavor. My boyfriend once told me not to drain the fat from the ground beef I had just browned because he thought I was throwing away all the flavor. After I picked myself up off the floor from laughing, I quickly explained to him that fat is not the only flavor that tastes good. There are so many spices available and many of them have positive effects on our health.

Salt and pepper go well with just about everything, but there is so much more out there to give your food a little (or a lot) of zing! Here is a list of just a few of the hundreds of spices on the market today.

Anise- has a licorice flavor- goes well with chicken or fish.

Fresh basil- goes great in salads, and pasta sauces.

Capers- give a salty, sour flavor. Excellent with fish and chicken.

Cayenne- very hot! Goes on anything you want to have a hot, spicy flavor.

Cinnamon– goes great on oatmeal, toast, yogurt or fruit.

Cumin– this one has a nice kick and goes well in chili, taco meat and beans.

Curry powder– great on chicken, fish, shrimp, scallops and vegetables.

Dill– goes great on salmon and eggs, or in yogurt as a dip.

Garlic– great on salads, chicken, fish, beef, pork, vegetables, soups or stews.

Ginger– adds a nice zip to soups, poultry or seafood.

Horseradish– gives your beef a real kick!

Lemon– really gives great flavor to seafood, chicken, salads, beans, vegetables and even water

Mint– nice on vegetables and in tea or sparkling water.

Mustard– goes well on chicken and salmon or in a salad dressing.

Onion– include in soups, stews, sauces, fish, beef, poultry, and eggs.

Oregano– has an "Italian" flavor.

Parsley– top your fish, poultry, eggs, vegetables and salad.

Rosemary– great in barley and baked poultry.

Tarragon– excellent on fish, beef and vegetables.

Turmeric– adds an Indian flavor and color

Fat is a vital nutrient that keeps our bodies working correctly. Fat not only provides energy for the body, it is an important building block in making hormones, controlling inflammation, and aids in absorption of vitamins and minerals. We've always been taught to avoid fat. We all went on low fat diets and thought we were doing ourselves a favor, but we weren't losing weight. Why? Because so many of the low fat foods on the market took out fat but added sugar. Next time you're in the store, look at the label of a no fat cookie or other product. You'll see that the added sugar also means you're still getting a lot of calories. The bottom line is calories still count. A gram of fat has more than twice as many calories as a gram of protein or carbohydrate. I would encourage you to incorporate certain fats in your diet, but choose wisely. We are looking for monounsaturated and polyunsaturated fats. Olive and coconut oils are my favorite. They have lots of antioxidants which contain anti-aging properties and it will also help you feel full. Just don't use olive oil for cooking. When using high heat, use coconut, grape seed, peanut or safflower oils, or even a cooking spray like Pam works well.

Walnuts, salmon and flaxseeds are also a great choice; they are packed with omega three's for a healthy heart. Almonds and avocados are healthy choices as well. Moderation is the key here. Fats are packed with calories, so a small handful of nuts, a tablespoon of olive oil, or one-fourth of an avocado is all you will need.

Having these good fats before a meal will send a signal to the brain that you are full and this will help in your weight loss efforts.

Tips on fat:

+ Avoid- trans fat, why? Because trans fat raises LDL or bad cholesterol and lowers the good cholesterol, which puts you at risk for heart disease and diabetes. Trans fat is in shortening, some margarine, crackers candies cookies, snack foods, baked goods and processed foods. According to the American Heart Association you should have less than two grams per day.

+ Consider fish. Most fish are lower in saturated fat than meat. It also has the good fats that help your body not store fat.

+ When eating out, always ask what types of oils are used or how things are cooked.

+ Always read your ingredient list. If you see words like hydrogenated, or partially hydrogenated, shortening, or palm kernel oil, you know it will contain at least some trans fat. Instead, go for natural oils like soybean, coconut oil, palm fruit or olive oils.

+ Go for omega three essential fatty acids: salmon, tuna, swordfish, flaxseed, walnuts, seaweed, or sardines. These will also have an anti-inflammatory effect on your body.

+ Omega six has a pro-inflammatory effect. This doesn't mean we don't need them, because we do, it just means we need a better balance of omega threes and sixes. Omega sixes are found in vegetable oil and some meats.

+ Nuts are good for you, but be aware that a cup of nuts will contain about 70 grams of fat. Stick to a single serving.

+ Going totally fat free is not your friend. Be sure to include good fats. Bet you never thought you'd hear your weight loss coach say "include" fat. For example, instead of mayo (bad fat), choose avocado, or olive oil. Instead of regular cheese, go for nut cheese; Instead of whole eggs, use egg whites and add avocado or ground flaxseeds; instead of butter, choose olive oil. When choosing dairy, go for the fat free. Add walnuts or ground flaxseed for the "good" fat in your meal.

+ The general rule is that if the fat comes from a plant source, it's going to be a better choice than an animal source. That said, avoid vegetable oil.

Other fats:

Oil of any kind, one tablespoon
Anything fried (crispy)
Butter, one pat
Visible fat on meats or chicken skin
Egg yolks. (Not saying these are bad, just count them as your fat, and have no more than two.)
Cheese, any kind
Dairy products that aren't labeled fat free like cream, cottage cheese, sour cream or yogurt
★Salad dressing

★Most foods labeled non fat or fat free, usually have added sugar. This is why it's so important to see what's in your food on your ingredient lists.

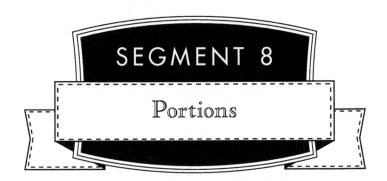

SEGMENT 8

Portions

PORTIONS ARE THE key to success, specifically with certain food groups, like carbs, fats and proteins. As for your green veggies, they fall under the "all you can eat" category, so load up on those. For the rest, keep your portions in check. It's not always practical to think that you can weigh every food you put on your plate. What you can do, however, is learn to recognize what key serving sizes look like, to help you know the right amount to serve yourself or eat at a restaurant. Your portion for carbs should always be one serving or less.

✦ Get a small, inexpensive scale so you can see what 4 oz. looks like.

✦ Use the same size plates and bowls at each meal so that you can get use to what proper portion sizes look like on each dish.

✦ Be sure to use smaller plates than the ones you are used to. Now you can have a full plate and not feel deprived.

✦ Develop visual cues by matching portion sizes to familiar items.

> A three oz. serving of meat is the size of a deck of cards or a bar of soap. It's ok to do a little more for the protein category. I usually have about 6 oz.

> ½ -cup of brown rice would just about fill a regular-sized cupcake wrapper

> One ounce of cheese is about the size of four dice. That's more than enough! I'm not a fan of dairy fat but this is just FYI so if you find yourself at the party cheese platter you know where to stop.

> A portion of meat or chicken should be the size and thickness of your palm

> One cup of oatmeal= your fist

> ½ of a cup cooked pasta = the size of half of a baseball

> A handful of nuts should be no bigger than a small egg

✦ Sandwich meat should be equivalent to the thickness of one standard slice of bread. Vegetables should be twice the thickness of the meat.

✦ Eyeball food portions based on the amount of room they take up on a dinner plate. For example, on an eight inch plate, half of the plate should be covered with vegetables, one-fourth with a low GI carb, and one-fourth (or more) with a protein. with a sprinkle of fat. Focus mostly on filling the plate with veggies and protein and a little fat often leaving the carbs out and your body will become inefficient at storing fat! You do need carbs, but not at every meal, especially not later in the day.

Once you see these a few times it will become second nature. Go easy on yourself; you are looking for progress not perfection.

★★Remember veggies are on the all you can eat list but you are choosing <u>one serving </u>from the carb, fat, and protein categories. It's very important to know those serving sizes. If you are still hungry, go back for seconds on the veggies or maybe even the protein, just be mindful of having more than one serving of carbs per meal!

To review portions:

Protein –

The goal would be to aim for at least 20 to 25 grams per meal

→ All meats, chicken, fish, or seafood- four to six ounces

→ Eggs – two whole with two whites (eggs have six grams of protein per egg, with four grams in the white. If you want your fat to come from a different source, omit the yolks and go for five whites)

→ Cottage cheese or yogurt ¾ cup

Carbs

→ Rice, beans, split peas, peas, quinoa, oatmeal (dry), or pasta -½ cup

→ Yam or sweet potato – one small

→ Low glycemic bread – one slice

→ Fruit- one medium or ¾ cup of berries

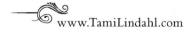

Fat

→ Oils (any) -one tablespoon

→ Nuts – small handful

→ Avocado- ¼

→ Hummus – two tablespoons

Veggies-

Are free so enjoy them! The non starchy kind of course.

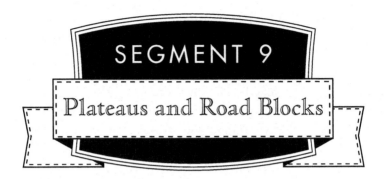

SEGMENT 9

Plateaus and Road Blocks

HOW DO YOU know if you plateau? A true plateau is when you have no fat loss, no inches lost, and no weight loss. If you are losing inches but not weight, this is not a plateau which means you are losing fat. You are still on the road to success. Most often when we diet, we lose weight, plateau and ultimately quit, then gain the weight back. I want a lifetime of success for you, so here are some tips:

1　Journaling
　　a.　*Continue to journal.*
　　　　Write down the foods you eat and the quantity: breakfast, lunch, dinner and snacks. Look for patterns. Is sugar starting to creep back in on a regular basis? Are you going back for seconds making your portions too big? The only way this will work is if you are totally honest. This is your life, your health and your weight loss success. Journaling is a great tool, and if you're honest it can really help you. It's also great practice in breaking down your foods in their categories of carbs, proteins, fats and veggies.

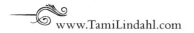
b. *Journal your exercise.*

Are you doing exactly the same thing you were doing five or six weeks ago? If so, kick it up a notch. Adding a little extra duration or intensity may be all you need. Are the excuses coming more frequently to not exercise at all? How many days are you working out, and for how long? Are you continuing to challenge yourself?

2   **Maybe it's time for another detox.**

If you are in a plateau, another way to get back on track, besides checking in with your eating and exercise is to detox again. Now that you're using your journal, maybe some of those addicting carbs or refined sugars are creeping their way back in more than you thought and it's time to get them "out of your system".

2   **Re-read your vision!**

Make sure you are re-reading your vision both in the morning and just before you go to bed. This helps tell your subconscious that you are not giving up and what it is that you really want. You may want to revise it or add more details on what it is that you really want. Be sure to visualize this as though it has already happened.

Questions to ask yourself:

1   Do you have a "never again" attitude? Are you really fed up with the old you? If not, it's time to get "mad". Start by remembering why you bought this book. How did you feel then?

2   How can you make this something you are aim-
    ing toward, rather than something you are running
    from? Think about what you are focusing on. Make
    it your vision!

3   What do you really, really want? What is your vision
    for your life and health?

4   Are you doing things that support what you real-
    ly want? Are you reading your labels? Do you keep
    junk foods out of the house?

5   Have you begun to change your limiting beliefs?
    Start by going to the internet to find out how dan-
    gerous sugar is or how wonderful asparagus is. You
    will begin to believe something different about them
    both if you do.

6   Are you setting yourself up to win – setting easy
    to reach "short term "goals to go toward your big-
    ger goals? Easy things like planning dinner. Do you
    have dinner planned or will you wing it when you
    get hungry later?

7   Are you surrounding yourself with people that sup-
    port you or people that are like minded? If not, it's
    time to set boundaries.

8   Do you catch yourself sabotaging your own goals?
    Are you still buying cookies "for the kids"? Don't
    keep this stuff in the house! Make it a special treat
    to go out any buy that one cookie at the specialty
    shop. You will also be teaching them that cookies

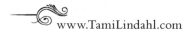

are a treat not an everyday occurrence. Win, win, just sayin… ☺

Take a good long look at these questions; write about them, how you feel and the solutions will come. There may be times you are uncomfortable with them, but that means growth is about to happen, so embrace it. Taking that hard look in the mirror is tough, but you will get through it and you will grow and learn. I tell my fitness clients: "if it doesn't kill you, it will make you stronger!"

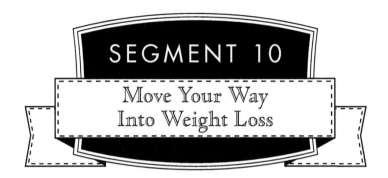

SEGMENT 10

Move Your Way
Into Weight Loss

Cardio.

A CARDIO WORKOUT SIMPLY means moving your body enough to increase your heart rate. You want to aim for 220-your age x 80%= target heart rate or beats per minute (bpm). Frankly, that's way too much math for me so a simpler formula would be 180- your age = your goal bpms. So if you are 50 it would be 180-50= 130 bpm. Be sure to listen to your body! If your heart feels like it's going to jump out your chest or you can hardly talk, then you are over doing it and you need to slow down; don't sit down, just slow down. I would recommend that you work up to keeping your target bpm's for 45 minutes to an hour but you definitely don't have to start with that much. For a beginner, if five minutes is all you can do, then start there. Another way to get more of a workout in if you are new is to split it up. If all you can do is five minutes, then do five minutes, but then add another five minutes later on in that same day and it will still equal 10 minutes of cardio. Continue to bump it up adding one or two minutes on each side and before you know it you'll be able to get 30 minutes in by simply moving your body 15 minutes twice a day. Eventually you'll work up to 30 continuous minutes for more endurance, but this is a doable way to start. Cardio also brings out the endorphins in us (the feel-good hormones). So, even if you don't like the exercise, I promise that you will love the way you feel when you finish! No one ever left my gym wishing they hadn't been there!

As with anything that you know you need to do, you have to include your cardio workout in your weekly planner. As women, we are so busy that if it's not in our planner, it won't get done. Make sure you are including cardio at least three days a week. Five or six would be better but for someone new, but three days is a great place to start.

If you are a non- exerciser and you get moving, the weight will fall off. I recommend seeking the advice of a personal trainer or taking classes so you can ask questions of the instructor.

Ok, with that said, it takes 3500 calories to gain or lose a pound. So, if you eat an extra 3500 calories, you'll gain a pound and if you burn an extra 3500 you'll lose a pound. Don't panic, I don't mean it has to be done in one day. If you burn an extra 500 calories a day for a week that equals 3500 and there is your pound lost. Here is a list of things you can so to get moving, and losing:

- Bicycling, stationary vigorous, 756 – moderate, 504
- Jump rope, 720
- Circuit training, 576
- Beach volleyball, 576
- Kickboxing, 540
- Aerobics, step or high impact, 504
- Row machine – moderate pace 504
- Hiking, 414
- Golf, 396 (no cart, of course)
- Walking briskly, 360
- Tae kwon do, 342

These calculations are based on 60 minutes and a person that weighs 150lbs and are approximate.

There are so many other things from dancing to housework that are considered cardio. As long as you monitor your heart rate you'll know if you're doing enough.

Resistance training

Many women think resistance or strength training is for men only, but that could not be farther from the truth. It is extremely important for us as well for several reasons. For weight loss purposes, as I have said in earlier chapters, "muscle dictates metabolism." The more lean muscle we have, the more efficient our calorie-burning capabilities are. If you want your body to be in a fat-burning mode, this is the way to do it. Think of it as cardio burns calories now and resistance burns calories the rest of the day- we need both! Some of my clients have expressed concern with "bulking up," but as women we don't have the hormones that would create big muscles, and we are not talking about spending 6 hours in the gym every day, which is what it would take to look like those women on the cover of Muscle magazine. I am talking about using light weights with more reps. You may feel after just a couple of workouts that your muscles are bulking, but they are just swelling, so don't give up. You will be better in the long run for having done it.

Another very important reason for resistance training is that it will help you build your bone density. This is why women start getting osteoporosis sooner than men. Men naturally have more muscle mass which is also why more women struggle with weight more than men. This doesn't mean men can't be affected by osteoporosis or weight issues, they just tend to have the advantage over women because of their tendency to have more muscle.

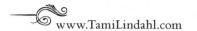

After working a particular muscle group, I recommend waiting at least 48 hours before working that same group again. For example you could work chest and triceps Monday, back and biceps Tuesday. You don't need to hit the chest again until Wednesday or Thursday.

Interval training is probably one of the best forms of exercise for weight loss. This is when you get your heart rate up really high, then recover. Then do that again. Circuit training can do that and it's a great bang for your buck because you can get some cardio in and strength training in at the same time.

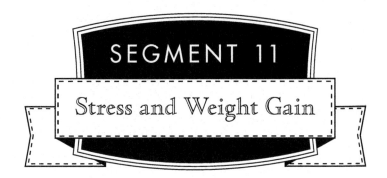

SEGMENT 11

Stress and Weight Gain

HORMONES HAVE A big part in weight loss or weight gain. There are several ways in which stress can contribute to weight gain as well. When we are under chronic stress, whether it's work-related, family or even physical stress, our bodies trigger a release of a hormone called cortisol. Here are a few reasons why stress and cortisol create weight gain:

1   Cortisol actually slows down your metabolism and tells your body to store fat. Particularly around the mid section, also known as "belly fat". Not only is it undesirable to look at, it's more dangerous to your health than fat that gets stored in other parts of the body.

2   Chronic stress can alter blood sugar levels, which you know can lead to weight gain, however, it can also cause fatigue and mood swings. Additionally, it has been linked to metabolic syndrome, which can lead to all kinds of health problems, including heart disease and diabetes.

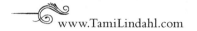

3   Craving the wrong foods. When you get stressed out, do you reach for the tub of ice cream or other sugary, salty or processed foods? This is typical, so if you are stressed out all the time, you can see where this will lead you. If you are living a stressed life-style, chances are you will run to the fast food places more often and again, this can result in you eating too much of the processed junk foods.

So, what can you do?

You can't just change jobs (or heck, maybe you can) or get rid of your family (although at times, you may want to). Here are some tips to handle stress so it doesn't handle you!

1   **Get your exercise in!** Exercise is a great stress reliev-er, from punching and kicking your way through a kickboxing class, to resistance training to stretching to yoga. Yoga is an awesome way to get rid of stress because it's about moving your way into stillness. You can use NET (no extra time) to de-stress and workout at the same time! Yoga is also about stretch-ing which is an awesome stress reducer to your mind and your body.

2   **Breathe.** Have you ever noticed that you are sit-ting at your computer and realize you aren't real-ly breathing? Every hour or so stop and take some deep breaths. In through your nose and out your mouth. Listen to the sound of the breath, and feel your chest expand as you inhale. Just several cycles of breathe can make a real difference and only takes a few minutes.

3   **Music can have a huge effect on our moods and stress levels.** You may enjoy Gun's n' Roses or Aerosmith but any head banging won't do you any favors if you are stressed out. Instead try listening something a little softer (there is a reason spas play the music that they do). If you are a die hard rock and roller at least listen to the music that makes you feel really good. No sad songs or songs that bring back unpleasant memories, just happy, feel good songs.

4   **Take time for yourself.** I know as women we have jobs or kids and very busy lives, so it can sometimes feel unnatural to take time for ourselves. Getting a massage or pedicure is always nice but also mean things like doing the things you like to do, like gardening (which can include family...or not) taking up an instrument, writing, arts & crafts, or anything that makes you feel good about yourself and puts a smile on your face.

These are some little things you can do to relieve stress and stay on the road to fitness. It may seem silly and you may be thinking: "How can a pedicure help me lose weight?" But, if you take even half the advice from this action guide, you will see lasting results, because these are all just little pieces to the puzzle!

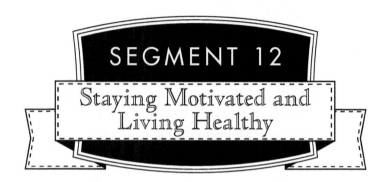

SEGMENT 12

Staying Motivated and Living Healthy

Celebrate!

YOU DID IT! Some sections may have been easy and some, not so much, but you did it. Take your pictures now and please send them to me, and with your permission, I would love to share them to help inspire others.

It takes some effort to stay on track with eating right and continuing your exercise. It's so easy to get comfortable or complacent and before you know it, slowly but surely the weight creeps back on. Whether it's some dessert items that someone brings home and now you have dessert three nights in a row. Someone brings donuts to the office and you "have just one," but it happens several times a week; you must pay attention. I'd hate to see you have all the success you wanted only to gain it back because you reached your goal so now you're "done." We are never done. Living a healthy lifestyle has so many benefits, including keeping it off!

Here are some tips:

1   Journal! Yes I know you've finished the program (but even if you still have more weight to lose) by continuing to journal, and writing down the cookies

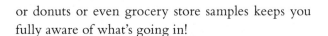

or donuts or even grocery store samples keeps you fully aware of what's going in!

2   **Read** something about of weight loss, eating low glycemic or exercise, **daily!** Reading something daily reinforces what you have learned or gives you new info on the subject and keeps you on TOMA- top of mind awareness. This really helps keep you on track and making the right choices. The more you read, whether is just a quick article you found online or getting through another book, the more easily eating right will be. It will also help make it much harder to eat the wrong foods because you will be very aware the consequences, and knowing how high glycemic or how much bad fat is in something makes it a lot harder so enjoy, so more often than not, you will find you just don't want those thing as much Again, this must be done **daily**. This exer- cise will strengthen your "attitude muscle" making it easier to make your best choices more often.

3   **Try new recipes.** Enjoying new ideas on different things you can eat makes living a healthy lifestyle enjoyable and will be something you can stick with forever. You will also be focusing on food that you can eat which makes eating right a positive experi- ence. Again, making this something you want to do forever.

4   **Get enough sleep!** Lack of sleep can affect your performance (physically or mentally), tears down your immune system, it can affect your mood (may- be that's just me), but it can also cause weight gain.

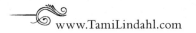

When you are really tired you tend to crave "comfort foods" which are not always your best choice.

5   **Try new ways to stay active.** Going to the gym is great and you should continue to go several times a week. Try a new class at the gym or change your routine so you continue to challenge your body. Go from boot camp to yoga. These are opposite types of workout and will keep you from getting bored. Sign up for a dance class, or join a sports team. Once you've paid and your team is counting on you, you'll show up.

6   **Continue to do your affirmations.** Find new ones, or continue with the ones that really get you motivated. Go on gratitude walks (or runs). As you walk or jog, go through all the things you are grateful for and say thank you. If you can do it out loud even better. It will bring more emotional intensity to it and give you the juice you need for the day!

7   **Always go organic.** With all the pesticides, antibiotics and hormones put on crops and feed to animals, going organic is very important. There is more and more evidence that these are affecting our health, our weight and our children! It may cost more, but really do you want to eat that chicken that's been fed corn laced with arsenic?

8   **Go green.** Keeping non-toxic household cleaners is also a great way to stay healthy. Most household cleaners have chemicals in them that have been linked to certain cancers and other childhood

diseases. When you are toxic, your liver has to work harder and has a harder time metabolizing fat.

Keep up the good work and continue in your journey. I'd love to hear from you to see your progress and answer more questions if you have them. Send your emails, stories, and pictures Tami@thinkFitwithTami.com

Tami Lindahl
http://www.FreeTrainerTips.com

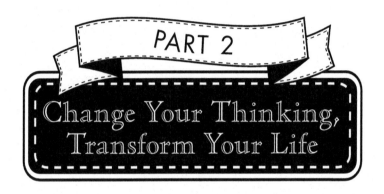

PART 2

Change Your Thinking,
Transform Your Life

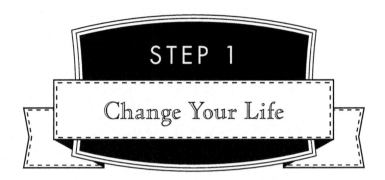

STEP 1

Change Your Life

Get the fire burning!

THE FIRST STEP to making changes in your life, whether its weight loss, business, or something in your personal life, is to be uncomfortable.. When we are comfortable, we don't do anything to make the changes that we know we "should" make. If something bothers you a little, it's not going to be enough to get you moving. It's only when we experience so much pain, that we even think about making changes. It's at that point we look at what it takes to make the changes and become willing to go to any length to get results we want. You must have a "never again" or " I can't take it anymore" attitude to keep you persevering, and keep you getting to the gym and making healthy food choices consistently! Reminding yourself (daily) of why you will continue to follow the advice of your weight loss coach will give you the burning desire that you will need to get you though, and will put that fire under your pants!

Now, once you've reached your goals, you may begin to feel comfortable again. This is often why people gain their weight back. You now have to switch gears and recognize the pleasure of what it is to have reached your goals, feel

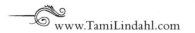

awesome, and fit into your skinny jeans again. So it all starts with acknowledging your pain, using it to fuel your motivation, and then basking in the pleasure of your results.... Being truly grateful (daily) for your health is the best way to accomplish that!

I asked you to create a vision at the beginning of this book. You could also create a vision of your life a year from now if you DON'T lose the weight. What does that look like? What does that feel like? Bring lots of detail to this one too. The more you see how uncomfortable you are, the more willing you will become to taking the actions to change. We don't do anything to change until we are uncomfortable enough. The pain of staying the same must be greater than the pain of change....

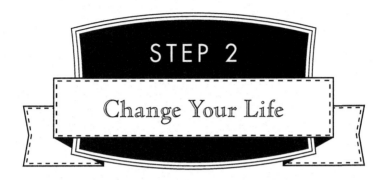

STEP 2

Change Your Life

Make a decision and move toward it!

THE FIRST PART of this step is to make a real decision. You must decide right here, right now what you want, and tell yourself that you will go to any length to get it. If you have decided that you want to lose weight, all the choices for the rest of the day, week, or month will come easily. If you have truly decided that losing weight and getting healthy is what you want, then you will skip the fries, write in your journal, and go to the gym, even though you don't "feel like it." Procrastination is the opposite of decision, so if you find yourself saying, "I'll do my work-out tomorrow," you'll know you are on a slippery slope.

> "A real decision is measured by the fact that you have taken new action. If there is no action, then you truly haven't decided."
> –Tony Robbins

Now that you have made the decision, you must look toward your goal, and not away from something else. If your issue is weight, for example, you must look forward to a leaner healthier you, and not away from being fat. If you

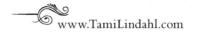

are running away from something you are still focusing on the thing you don't want, like in this example, fat. You get more of what you focus on. I hear so many clients say they put their "fat" picture right on the fridge to remind them of how fat they are and to not eat so much… this is the kiss of death to success. Instead, put a picture of a healthier version of you so you see daily what you are working toward, not what you are running away from. This works with all areas in your life. Need money? Don't run from lack, run to abundance. Need a mate? Don't run from loneliness, run toward friendship and love.

So what are you moving toward? Let's start with your goals you wrote in the beginning of the book. Keep a close eye on them. Keeping records of your success is the key because you can "see" your progress right there on paper. Yes, you will see it in the mirror and in the way your clothes fit, but, seeing the numbers of inches, fat and weight is a powerful tool in keeping you on track. That's why I have you measure yourself every three weeks, it's enough time to see your numbers change but not so far apart that you lose sight of these goals. Looking forward to measurements will really help you in your success.

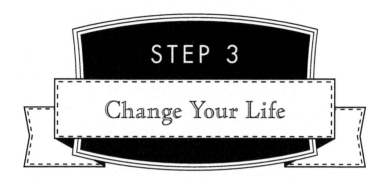

STEP 3

Change Your Life

Think yourself thin!

YOU MAY HAVE heard the expression "thoughts are things." I believe this is true, and here's why: Anything you have EVER done began with a thought. Have you ever accomplished something that you were proud of? I'm sure you have, but you didn't get there without thinking about it first. It's time now to use your imagination. Imagine what your life would be like if you lost weight. What would be different for you? Would you have more success either personally or professionally? Would you have your self-esteem back? More romance? These are questions you may ask yourself, but I bring these questions up because I want you to get your creative juices flowing. I want you to be able to begin to "picture" your life how you want it. See yourself there. Think yourself thin.

> "Nothing happens unless we first dream."
> – Carl Sandburg

You have already created your vision, but another exercise you can do here is to create a vision board. Create a poster or a board with images of things you want to see come into

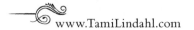
your life. Images of what you think being thin or healthy means to you. For example, pictures of people being active, pictures of you at the weight you want to be (and if you don't have any, put your head on the body you want), pictures of successful people, or maybe if romance is what you want, then put those up there too. Remember, this is your life, so what (or who) do you want to be in it? Put images of things that make you feel good. This process is just part of the journey and if you don't feel good in the journey you won't feel good when you get there and your results won't last!!

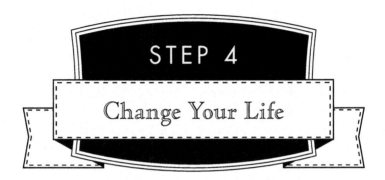

STEP 4

Change Your Life

Get out your MAP!

YOU KNOW WHAT you want and where you want to go, so how do you get there?

It's time to get out your **MAP**....
Massive **A**ction **P**lan, that is.

You got uncomfortable enough and now you have that burning desire to want to do something different (step one). You are moving toward your goal (step two). You see yourself thin (step three), but now you must have a plan and you must take action! If losing weight is your goal, ask yourself what you need to do to make it happen. This program is a great start! But wait, having a plan is just not enough! You have your gym schedule lined up, you have your daily menu planned for the next week but if there is no action on your part, you won't reach your goal. It will take consistent, committed action daily, to see real results! Your actions are to get on your weekly calls or meeting with your trainer as scheduled, plan out your meals, and exercise, journal daily, and work the other nine steps! So, get out your MAP, head toward your goals, and change your life!

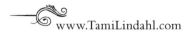

There are also actions I want you to NOT take. As you begin your new way of life you will begin to notice how you "talk to yourself." What are you telling yourself? Did you give yourself an "at-a-boy" for showing up to the gym, or did you put yourself down because you didn't stay long enough or do enough? Just begin to listen to what you are saying to yourself. Awareness is the 1st step toward making your positive changes. You can't change something you are unaware of!! As you notice the negative talk, do something, anything, to change your pattern. Jump up and down, run to a mirror and make funny faces. It really doesn't matter but this will begin to stop you in your tracks of continuing a habit that might be as old as you! This takes practice and you will have to do it over and over again, but it works as long as you never give up!

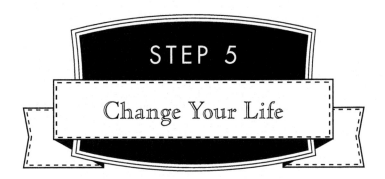

STEP 5

Change Your Life

Faith and affirmations

YOU MUST BELIEVE you can do it. You must believe you can get the results you want and you must believe you can maintain your healthy lifestyle. But, how do you do that when you have tried so many other diets or weight loss programs, only to gain the weight back and perhaps more? In step two I talked about visualizing ourselves thin. That is the first part of getting the faith you need. If your self-esteem is down, it may be very challenging to truly believe this will work for you. So, start with your visualizations. See yourself the way you want and feel how it feels to have achieved it. Then go to your affirmations. Affirmations are a very powerful tool that can really help you with getting your mindset in the right place. You may feel silly doing it, but as I tell my clients: "Hear me now believe me later."

Here is how it works: you pick one or two and say them over and over, with as much emotional intensity as you can muster. I recommend you do it in the morning because it will set the tone for the whole day! I recommend you start with doing this for just a few minutes, perhaps the entire length of your shower or while blow drying your hair, then

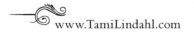
work up to doing these incantations or affirmations for an hour, during your workout maybe.

Use one of these or make one of your own:

✦   I visualize my future and I'm so excited about it.

✦   Life gets easier and easier.

✦   Nothing tastes as good as skinny feels.

✦   Today I honor my body.

✦   I deserve to be happy and successful.

✦   I have the power to change myself.

✦   I can forgive and understand others and their motives.

✦   At last, at last I've broken free and won. Now it's time to love myself and really have some fun!

✦   I deserve to be loved.

✦   I can do this!

✦   Today, I am raising my standards for myself.

✦   I can make my own choices and decisions.

✦   Today, I choose to be responsible, and NOT a victim.

✦   I can choose happiness whenever I wish no matter what my circumstances.

✦   I am flexible and open to change in every aspect of my life.

✦ I act with confidence having a general plan and accept plans are open to alteration.

✦ It is enough to have done my best.

✦ I don't eat like that anymore.

What you feed your mind is as important as what you feed your body! What images do you see? What words are you saying, to yourself or even out loud?

This is why "diet" or most exercise programs work only temporarily. People may change their food, and they may change the way they move their bodies. If they don't change the way they think, they will end up right back where they started. These affirmations are a start. When you hear yourself say "I can't do this" change it immediately to something more positive, like, "I'm not giving up!"

Remember, YOU are the only one who can control your thoughts; no one else can do this for you. By feeding your mind more positive words and images you will begin to see changes and the results you have been wanting for a long time!

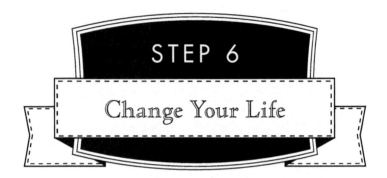

STEP 6

Change Your Life

Getting real, and changing your limiting beliefs.

WHAT DO YOU believe about exercise, eating right, yourself, or following through with the things you know you should be doing? Do you find yourself rationalizing why you don't work-out? Maybe you tell yourself you don't have time, or it's too far. Maybe you even believe that going to a gym is embarrassing or you feel lost or don't know what to do when you get there. Sound familiar? What is your story you tell yourself to justify why you are not eating the foods you know will bring you closer to your goals? Perhaps it was: "I was starving so I just had to eat something," "my family won't eat like that," or "I didn't want to make someone feel bad," or "I just can't resist cheesecake". Well guess what? These are just glorified excuses! These are things you tell yourself and for the most part, you really believe them. So, what you must do now is to change that limiting belief, so you begin to tell yourself the truth.

It's time to change your story. You are the author of your life and you have the power to change your story. Here is an exercise to get you started:

1   Get a sheet of paper and make two columns. In column one, write down all the stories you tell yourself. Be honest! It's all about getting real and getting really honest with yourself. Make this list as long as you want, the more the better!

2   In the second column write the opposing belief. So if your limiting belief is "I have never been able to keep the weight off before, what makes me think this time is different?" The opposing belief would be " today is a new day and I have the power to change my life and my habits" "I don't have time" then the opposing belief is "I put my workouts in my planner so it's part of my schedule." Or, if you believe "I just can't resist cheesecake" the opposing belief would be "I choose only foods that bring me closer to my goals" or "I don't eat that stuff anymore."

3   To embed these new beliefs in your brain, try adding them to your morning affirmations. This will really help drive this home to your subconscious. This is something you should do DAILY! Keep your brain on track with what you say you want.

If you are still finding this difficult, go back to step one, and find your burning desire to change the way you think about exercise and eating right.

Another great way to change your beliefs about food or exercise is to read something EVERYDAY about what you want more of. For example, you know you "should" eat more veggies so go to the internet, everyday, and search for benefits of your favorite veggies. When these articles talk

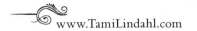

about how great they are for you, and you do this every day you will begin to be more attracted to eating them.

This sounds like a lot of work but it only takes a few minutes. Write down your top 6 favorite vegetables and look one up a day for a week (yes you can take Sunday off... but why?) This should take you less than 5 minutes a day but I can promise if you do this for at least 21 days you have a whole different belief about veggies and you will **WANT** to eat more of them.

This includes looking up recipes too so you can kill two birds with one stone, reinforce your belief system to healthy thinking and end up with some great recipes of things you like.

The bottom line is **Belief = Behavior = results.** If you believe a certain food is good for you (emotionally of physically) your belief will lead you to wanting it. We all know if you are eating certain foods you will see certain results. The idea here is to believe good things about your best choices and bad things about bad choices.

When you do your daily mental conditioning, by searching the internet for example, your thoughts about certain foods change and you *naturally* begin to eat differently. For me doing this exercise when I wrote my 1st book, I looked at potatoes in a whole new light. They used to be my friend and my comfort, now they are the enemy and I have embedded in my head if I eat that I will get fat". Now I have also attached a very negative association with being fat so it's a rare day that I go for potatoes!

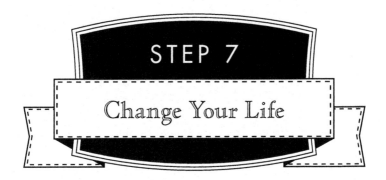

STEP 7

Change Your Life

Prayer, meditation and gratitude.

Prayer is a powerful tool in creating the life you want. Not just for weight loss but in all aspects. To be clear, I'm not pushing religion by any stretch. I'm just talking about becoming more spiritual. I'm talking about having a relationship with a god of your understanding, your divine self, that inner voice that guides you. Pray to your higher power, not anyone else's. Turning your will over to the care of God as you understand him is, well, like magic you will begin to see amazing things happen in your life. Just be mindful of what you are asking for. Ask for guidance and strength to get you through your day, not "dear God, why can't I lose weight?" Ask what you can do, today, to move closer to our goals.

When asking for guidance and strength, quiet yourself, and the answers will come. Meditation is all about listening. I know it's hard to even be still for a minute, so this will take practice, maybe years, before you are really able to be still in your mind. But, remember, this is about progress not perfection!

Being grateful is very important to your lasting success and just being fulfilled in general. Personally, I include my

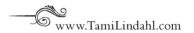

"thank-you's" in my morning prayers, but a gratitude list is powerful too. Make a list, every day, of at least 10 things you are grateful for and be sure to include even the little things. Being grateful, for even a half-inch lost keeps you out of your head and can prevent you from having negative self-talk. Be thankful for all your health from healthy organs, the weight you lost, to the pants you now fit into, or even being grateful that you got out of bed this morning! I would also recommend you add other things or people in your life that you are grateful for! Maybe you are grateful for your job, supportive family, or this program and your weight loss coach.☺

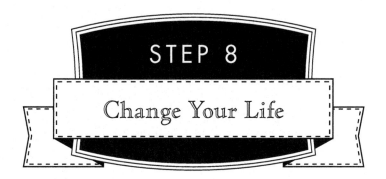

STEP 8

Change Your Life

Set yourself up for success!

You are well on your way! You have the desire you need to carry you through, you can imagine how great it will be, you have your map and you're moving toward your goals. You're even trying out that whole prayer thing. You are right on target. But let's make sure you set yourself up for success. Earlier on, you set your goals. Were they attainable? Did you set your goals too high to reach? Did you set a goal to work out everyday only to find you didn't work out at all? Did you set a goal of losing 10 lbs. a week? It may be time to revisit your goals so you don't end up discouraged, or worse, wanting to quit!

It's time now, to review and re-evaluate. If you are having trouble getting through the workouts, let's find out why. If the gym you joined is too far, you need to put another plan in place. If you just don't like to work out, begin charting how you feel after a workout? Do you feel energized, proud, tired hopeless, hopeful? Measure your emotion. Once you begin to see these feelings in writing, you will be more likely to workout. Same goes with your eating (which is why journaling is so important). How do you feel physically or

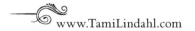

emotionally after finishing a bag of cookies or eating an order of fries? Again, seeing it in writing can lead to an "aha" moment.

Ok, with that said, this also applies to never letting yourself have a cookie or French Fries. These are occasional foods and this is a lifestyle, not a diet, so if you occasionally have it, don't beat yourself up. You are still doing great!

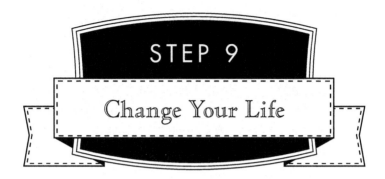

STEP 9

Change Your Life

Surround yourself with winners!

Have you ever noticed that people tend to associate with other people like themselves? Millionaires don't surround themselves with minimum wage workers, athletes don't mix with couch potatoes, and you don't see health nuts hanging out at the corner bar with a guy named Smokey Joe.

The best way to change your life and continue to grow and improve is to position yourself around others who are either experts in that area or others who are have similar goals. By doing this, you will have people around you who will encourage you, give positive advice, and help keep you on track.

If you hire a personal trainer that is so enthusiastic about health and fitness, it's bound to rub off on you. If you join an exercise class and you all decide to go somewhere after class, chances are, as a group, you will all make healthier food choices. When you are involved with a group trying to lose weight, the others will not only encourage you, they will expect more from you than you may expect from yourself. There is power in knowing you are helping and encouraging each other. One of our basic human needs is to contribute.

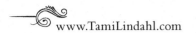

Same goes for the opposite. If you surround yourself with people that have unhealthy habits and don't have high standards, eventually it will rub off on you as well. I know that often times, you may be surrounded by family that may not have the best habits, but you love your family and choose your peers. Being an example to them is all you can do.

Staying "plugged in" to a group is your best route to lasting success. Just knowing that someone else cares about your success will keep you going.

> *"Most people's lives are a direct reflection of the expectations of their peer group."*
> *- Tony Robbins*

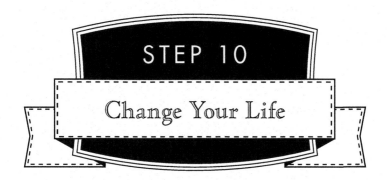

STEP 10

Change Your Life

Persistence...Never give up!

If you don't stick with something you will not be successful at it, right? As in the case with diets or weight loss programs, how many of them worked until you just gave up and went back to your old habits? All of them, or you wouldn't be here now. What those programs lack are the lessons on how to change your life and your mind on how you think about food and exercise. Persistence is forming a habit, and not giving up. These are habits you must adopt, daily.

1   You must go back to step one and look at what brings you here in the first place. What kind of pain will you be in (or stay in) if you don't follow through? What will your life be like if you go back to your old habits and continue to gain weight? Get that emotion and picture in your head! Read your visions daily.

2   Keep your vision and vision board where you can see them and focus on it daily.

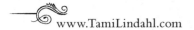

3   Keep your goals right in front of you so you know where you are and if you're on track, or not.

4   Make sure the action part of your MAP is in your schedule!

5   Don't skip your affirmations; this will help keep that negativity that creeps in and takes us down.

6   Ask your higher power for guidance and strength... You will get it!

7   Stay plugged in and continue with your support group, weight loss partner, trainer, or coach.

By now, hopefully some of these things are already habits, but write them down anyway... put it on your to do list. Do whatever it takes to incorporate these things in your life daily. The more persistent you are, the more success you'll have.

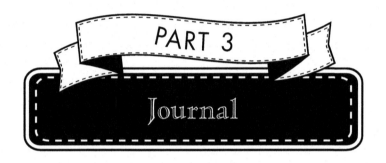

PART 3

Journal

Daily Journal

DAY 1

FOOD

BREAKFAST TIME

Protein_____

Fat_____

Veggies_____

Low GI Carb_____

SNACK TIME

Protein_____

Fat_____

Veggies_____

Low GI Carb_____

LUNCH TIME

Protein_____

Fat_____

Veggies_____

Low GI Carb_____

SNACK TIME

Protein_____

Fat_____

Veggies_____

Low GI Carb_____

DINNERTIME

Protein_____

Fat_____

Veggies_____

Low GI Carb_____

WATER

☐ ☐ ☐ ☐
☐ ☐ ☐ ☐

EXERCISE

Cardio_____

Strength_____

HOW DO YOU FEEL?

_____
_____
_____
_____
_____
_____
_____
_____
_____
_____
_____
_____
_____

QUOTE: Everything you want is out there waiting for you to ask. Everything you ever wanted, wants you. But you have to take action to get it.

~JACK CANFIELD

Daily Journal

DAY 2

FOOD

BREAKFAST TIME

Protein_____

Fat_____

Veggies_____

Low GI Carb_____

SNACK TIME

Protein_____

Fat_____

Veggies_____

Low GI Carb_____

LUNCH TIME

Protein_____

Fat_____

Veggies_____

Low GI Carb_____

SNACK TIME

Protein_____

Fat_____

Veggies_____

Low GI Carb_____

DINNERTIME

Protein_____

Fat_____

Veggies_____

Low GI Carb_____

WATER

☐ ☐ ☐ ☐
☐ ☐ ☐ ☐

EXERCISE

Cardio_____

Strength_____

HOW DO YOU FEEL?

_____
_____
_____
_____
_____
_____
_____
_____
_____
_____
_____
_____
_____
_____
_____
_____

AFFIRMATION: All I need is within me now.

Daily Journal

DAY 3

FOOD

BREAKFAST TIME

Protein_____

Fat_____

Veggies_____

Low GI Carb_____

SNACK TIME

Protein_____

Fat_____

Veggies_____

Low GI Carb_____

LUNCH TIME

Protein_____

Fat_____

Veggies_____

Low GI Carb_____

SNACK TIME

Protein_____

Fat_____

Veggies_____

Low GI Carb_____

DINNERTIME

Protein_____

Fat_____

Veggies_____

Low GI Carb_____

WATER

☐ ☐ ☐ ☐
☐ ☐ ☐ ☐

EXERCISE

Cardio_____

Strength_____

HOW DO YOU FEEL?

_____
_____
_____
_____
_____
_____
_____
_____
_____
_____
_____
_____
_____
_____
_____
_____

QUOTE: All things must change to something new, to something strange.

~HENRY WADSWORTH LONGFELLOW

Daily Journal

DAY 4

FOOD

BREAKFAST TIME

Protein_____

Fat_____

Veggies_____

Low GI Carb_____

SNACK TIME

Protein_____

Fat_____

Veggies_____

Low GI Carb_____

LUNCH TIME

Protein_____

Fat_____

Veggies_____

Low GI Carb_____

SNACK TIME

Protein_____

Fat_____

Veggies_____

Low GI Carb_____

DINNERTIME

Protein_____

Fat_____

Veggies_____

Low GI Carb_____

WATER

☐ ☐ ☐ ☐
☐ ☐ ☐ ☐

EXERCISE

Cardio_____

Strength_____

HOW DO YOU FEEL?

_____

_____

_____

_____

_____

_____

_____

_____

_____

_____

_____

_____

_____

_____

_____

_____

 HEALTH TIP: Now that you are detoxing your body, try detoxing your home. So many chemicals in your household cleaning products are linked to changes in hormones (which can lead to weight gain) and have other toxic effects on us.

Daily Journal

DAY 5

FOOD

BREAKFAST TIME

Protein_____

Fat_____

Veggies_____

Low GI Carb_____

SNACK TIME

Protein_____

Fat_____

Veggies_____

Low GI Carb_____

LUNCH TIME

Protein_____

Fat_____

Veggies_____

Low GI Carb_____

SNACK TIME

Protein_____

Fat_____

Veggies_____

Low GI Carb_____

DINNERTIME

Protein_____

Fat_____

Veggies_____

Low GI Carb_____

WATER

☐ ☐ ☐ ☐
☐ ☐ ☐ ☐

EXERCISE

Cardio_____

Strength_____

HOW DO YOU FEEL?

_____
_____
_____
_____
_____
_____
_____
_____
_____
_____
_____
_____
_____
_____
_____

QUOTE: All meaningful and lasting change starts first in your imagination and then works its way out. Imagination is more important than knowledge.

~ALBERT EINSTEIN

DAY 6

FOOD

BREAKFAST TIME

Protein_____

Fat_____

Veggies_____

Low GI Carb_____

SNACK TIME

Protein_____

Fat_____

Veggies_____

Low GI Carb_____

LUNCH TIME

Protein_____

Fat_____

Veggies_____

Low GI Carb_____

SNACK TIME

Protein_____

Fat_____

Veggies_____

Low GI Carb_____

DINNERTIME

Protein_____

Fat_____

Veggies_____

Low GI Carb_____

WATER

☐ ☐ ☐ ☐
☐ ☐ ☐ ☐

EXERCISE

Cardio_____

Strength_____

HOW DO YOU FEEL?

_____
_____
_____
_____
_____
_____
_____
_____
_____
_____
_____
_____
_____
_____

AFFIRMATION: I create new positive habits daily.

Daily Journal

DAY 7

FOOD

BREAKFAST TIME

Protein_____

Fat_____

Veggies_____

Low GI Carb_____

SNACK TIME

Protein_____

Fat_____

Veggies_____

Low GI Carb_____

LUNCH TIME

Protein_____

Fat_____

Veggies_____

Low GI Carb_____

SNACK TIME

Protein_____

Fat_____

Veggies_____

Low GI Carb_____

DINNERTIME

Protein_____

Fat_____

Veggies_____

Low GI Carb_____

WATER

☐ ☐ ☐ ☐
☐ ☐ ☐ ☐

EXERCISE

Cardio_____

Strength_____

HOW DO YOU FEEL?

_____
_____
_____
_____
_____
_____
_____
_____
_____
_____
_____
_____
_____
_____
_____

 HEALTH TIP: What's in your food? Always check your labels. Not just how many calories or fat, but where do they come from. Your ingredient list is very revealing!

Daily Journal

DAY 8

FOOD

BREAKFAST TIME

Protein_____

Fat_____

Veggies_____

Low GI Carb_____

SNACK TIME

Protein_____

Fat_____

Veggies_____

Low GI Carb_____

LUNCH TIME

Protein_____

Fat_____

Veggies_____

Low GI Carb_____

SNACK TIME

Protein_____

Fat_____

Veggies_____

Low GI Carb_____

DINNERTIME

Protein_____

Fat_____

Veggies_____

Low GI Carb_____

WATER

☐ ☐ ☐ ☐
☐ ☐ ☐ ☐

EXERCISE

Cardio_____

Strength_____

HOW DO YOU FEEL?

_____
_____
_____
_____
_____
_____
_____
_____
_____
_____
_____
_____
_____
_____
_____
_____
_____

QUOTE: Any change, even for the better, is always accompanied by drawbacks and discomforts.

~ARNOLD BENNETT

Daily Journal

DAY 9

FOOD

BREAKFAST TIME

Protein_____

Fat_____

Veggies_____

Low GI Carb_____

SNACK TIME

Protein_____

Fat_____

Veggies_____

Low GI Carb_____

LUNCH TIME

Protein_____

Fat_____

Veggies_____

Low GI Carb_____

SNACK TIME

Protein_____

Fat_____

Veggies_____

Low GI Carb_____

DINNERTIME

Protein_____

Fat_____

Veggies_____

Low GI Carb_____

WATER

☐ ☐ ☐ ☐
☐ ☐ ☐ ☐

EXERCISE

Cardio_____

Strength_____

HOW DO YOU FEEL?

_____
_____
_____
_____
_____
_____
_____
_____
_____
_____
_____
_____
_____
_____
_____
_____

 AFFIRMATION: I am so happy and grateful.

Daily Journal

DAY 10

FOOD

BREAKFAST TIME

Protein_____

Fat_____

Veggies_____

Low GI Carb_____

SNACK TIME

Protein_____

Fat_____

Veggies_____

Low GI Carb_____

LUNCH TIME

Protein_____

Fat_____

Veggies_____

Low GI Carb_____

SNACK TIME

Protein_____

Fat_____

Veggies_____

Low GI Carb_____

DINNERTIME

Protein_____

Fat_____

Veggies_____

Low GI Carb_____

WATER

☐ ☐ ☐ ☐
☐ ☐ ☐ ☐

EXERCISE

Cardio_____

Strength_____

HOW DO YOU FEEL?

_____
_____
_____
_____
_____
_____
_____
_____
_____
_____
_____
_____
_____
_____
_____

QUOTE: Have patience with all things, but chiefly have patience with yourself. Do not lose courage in considering your own imperfections but instantly set about remedying them - every day begin the task anew.

~SAINT FRANCIS DE SALES

Daily Journal

DAY 11

FOOD

BREAKFAST TIME

Protein_____

Fat_____

Veggies_____

Low GI Carb_____

SNACK TIME

Protein_____

Fat_____

Veggies_____

Low GI Carb_____

LUNCH TIME

Protein_____

Fat_____

Veggies_____

Low GI Carb_____

SNACK TIME

Protein_____

Fat_____

Veggies_____

Low GI Carb_____

DINNERTIME

Protein_____

Fat_____

Veggies_____

Low GI Carb_____

WATER

☐ ☐ ☐ ☐
☐ ☐ ☐ ☐

EXERCISE

Cardio_____

Strength_____

HOW DO YOU FEEL?

_____
_____
_____
_____
_____
_____
_____
_____
_____
_____
_____
_____
_____
_____
_____
_____

AFFIRMATION: Today I am raising my standards for myself.

Daily Journal
DAY 12

FOOD

BREAKFAST TIME

Protein_____

Fat_____

Veggies_____

Low GI Carb_____

SNACK TIME

Protein_____

Fat_____

Veggies_____

Low GI Carb_____

LUNCH TIME

Protein_____

Fat_____

Veggies_____

Low GI Carb_____

SNACK TIME

Protein_____

Fat_____

Veggies_____

Low GI Carb_____

DINNERTIME

Protein_____

Fat_____

Veggies_____

Low GI Carb_____

WATER

☐ ☐ ☐ ☐
☐ ☐ ☐ ☐

EXERCISE

Cardio_____

Strength_____

HOW DO YOU FEEL?

_____
_____
_____
_____
_____
_____
_____
_____
_____
_____
_____
_____
_____
_____
_____
_____

 HEALTH TIP: Having your gym bag packed and in the car ahead of time will help eliminate the temptation to "just skip it."

Daily Journal

DAY 13

FOOD

BREAKFAST TIME

Protein_____

Fat_____

Veggies_____

Low GI Carb_____

SNACK TIME

Protein_____

Fat_____

Veggies_____

Low GI Carb_____

LUNCH TIME

Protein_____

Fat_____

Veggies_____

Low GI Carb_____

SNACK TIME

Protein_____

Fat_____

Veggies_____

Low GI Carb_____

DINNERTIME

Protein_____

Fat_____

Veggies_____

Low GI Carb_____

WATER

☐ ☐ ☐ ☐
☐ ☐ ☐ ☐

EXERCISE

Cardio_____

Strength_____

HOW DO YOU FEEL?

_____
_____
_____
_____
_____
_____
_____
_____
_____
_____
_____
_____
_____
_____
_____
_____

 AFFIRMATION: I choose success, today.

Daily Journal

DAY 14

FOOD

BREAKFAST TIME

Protein_____

Fat_____

Veggies_____

Low GI Carb_____

SNACK TIME

Protein_____

Fat_____

Veggies_____

Low GI Carb_____

LUNCH TIME

Protein_____

Fat_____

Veggies_____

Low GI Carb_____

SNACK TIME

Protein_____

Fat_____

Veggies_____

Low GI Carb_____

DINNERTIME

Protein_____

Fat_____

Veggies_____

Low GI Carb_____

WATER

☐ ☐ ☐ ☐
☐ ☐ ☐ ☐

EXERCISE

Cardio_____

Strength_____

HOW DO YOU FEEL?

_____
_____
_____
_____
_____
_____
_____
_____
_____
_____
_____
_____
_____
_____
_____

 HEALTH TIP: Before reaching for butter or oils for added flavor, reach for spices or herbs. They can add a ton of flavor without all the fat and calories.

Daily Journal

DAY 15

FOOD

BREAKFAST TIME

Protein_____

Fat_____

Veggies_____

Low GI Carb_____

SNACK TIME

Protein_____

Fat_____

Veggies_____

Low GI Carb_____

LUNCH TIME

Protein_____

Fat_____

Veggies_____

Low GI Carb_____

SNACK TIME

Protein_____

Fat_____

Veggies_____

Low GI Carb_____

DINNERTIME

Protein_____

Fat_____

Veggies_____

Low GI Carb_____

WATER

☐ ☐ ☐ ☐
☐ ☐ ☐ ☐

EXERCISE

Cardio_____

Strength_____

HOW DO YOU FEEL?

_____
_____
_____
_____
_____
_____
_____
_____
_____
_____
_____
_____
_____
_____
_____
_____

 TO DO: Measure Today . . .

Daily Journal

DAY 16

FOOD

BREAKFAST TIME

Protein_____

Fat_____

Veggies_____

Low GI Carb_____

SNACK TIME

Protein_____

Fat_____

Veggies_____

Low GI Carb_____

LUNCH TIME

Protein_____

Fat_____

Veggies_____

Low GI Carb_____

SNACK TIME

Protein_____

Fat_____

Veggies_____

Low GI Carb_____

DINNERTIME

Protein_____

Fat_____

Veggies_____

Low GI Carb_____

WATER

☐ ☐ ☐ ☐
☐ ☐ ☐ ☐

EXERCISE

Cardio_____

Strength_____

HOW DO YOU FEEL?

_____
_____
_____
_____
_____
_____
_____
_____
_____
_____
_____
_____
_____
_____
_____

QUOTE: Miracles start to happen when you give as much energy to your dreams as you do your fears.

~RICHARD WILKINS

FOOD

BREAKFAST TIME

Protein_____

Fat_____

Veggies_____

Low GI Carb_____

SNACK TIME

Protein_____

Fat_____

Veggies_____

Low GI Carb_____

LUNCH TIME

Protein_____

Fat_____

Veggies_____

Low GI Carb_____

SNACK TIME

Protein_____

Fat_____

Veggies_____

Low GI Carb_____

DINNERTIME

Protein_____

Fat_____

Veggies_____

Low GI Carb_____

WATER

☐ ☐ ☐ ☐
☐ ☐ ☐ ☐

EXERCISE

Cardio_____

Strength_____

HOW DO YOU FEEL?

_____
_____
_____
_____
_____
_____
_____
_____
_____
_____
_____
_____
_____
_____
_____
_____

QUOTE: If we did all the things we were capable of, we would literally astound ourselves.

~THOMAS EDISON

Daily Journal

DAY 18

FOOD

BREAKFAST TIME

Protein_____

Fat_____

Veggies_____

Low GI Carb_____

SNACK TIME

Protein_____

Fat_____

Veggies_____

Low GI Carb_____

LUNCH TIME

Protein_____

Fat_____

Veggies_____

Low GI Carb_____

SNACK TIME

Protein_____

Fat_____

Veggies_____

Low GI Carb_____

DINNERTIME

Protein_____

Fat_____

Veggies_____

Low GI Carb_____

WATER

☐ ☐ ☐ ☐
☐ ☐ ☐ ☐

EXERCISE

Cardio_____

Strength_____

HOW DO YOU FEEL?

_____

_____

_____

_____

_____

_____

_____

_____

_____

_____

_____

_____

_____

AFFIRMATION: I am so grateful for my health.

Daily Journal

DAY 19

FOOD

BREAKFAST TIME

Protein_____

Fat_____

Veggies_____

Low GI Carb_____

SNACK TIME

Protein_____

Fat_____

Veggies_____

Low GI Carb_____

LUNCH TIME

Protein_____

Fat_____

Veggies_____

Low GI Carb_____

SNACK TIME

Protein_____

Fat_____

Veggies_____

Low GI Carb_____

DINNERTIME

Protein_____

Fat_____

Veggies_____

Low GI Carb_____

WATER

☐ ☐ ☐ ☐
☐ ☐ ☐ ☐

EXERCISE

Cardio_____

Strength_____

HOW DO YOU FEEL?

_____

_____

_____

_____

_____

_____

_____

_____

_____

_____

_____

_____

_____

_____

 HEALTH TIP: Choose whole beans instead of refried. They are not processed and are lower glycemic, and are often lower in saturated fat as well.

Daily Journal

DAY 20

FOOD

BREAKFAST TIME

Protein_____

Fat_____

Veggies_____

Low GI Carb_____

SNACK TIME

Protein_____

Fat_____

Veggies_____

Low GI Carb_____

LUNCH TIME

Protein_____

Fat_____

Veggies_____

Low GI Carb_____

SNACK TIME

Protein_____

Fat_____

Veggies_____

Low GI Carb_____

DINNERTIME

Protein_____

Fat_____

Veggies_____

Low GI Carb_____

WATER

☐ ☐ ☐ ☐
☐ ☐ ☐ ☐

EXERCISE

Cardio_____

Strength_____

HOW DO YOU FEEL?

_____
_____
_____
_____
_____
_____
_____
_____
_____
_____
_____
_____
_____
_____
_____

AFFIRMATION: I love my life. I am so blessed.

Daily Journal

DAY 21

FOOD

BREAKFAST TIME

Protein_____

Fat_____

Veggies_____

Low GI Carb_____

SNACK TIME

Protein_____

Fat_____

Veggies_____

Low GI Carb_____

LUNCH TIME

Protein_____

Fat_____

Veggies_____

Low GI Carb_____

SNACK TIME

Protein_____

Fat_____

Veggies_____

Low GI Carb_____

DINNERTIME

Protein_____

Fat_____

Veggies_____

Low GI Carb_____

WATER

☐ ☐ ☐ ☐
☐ ☐ ☐ ☐

EXERCISE

Cardio_____

Strength_____

HOW DO YOU FEEL?

_____

_____

_____

_____

_____

_____

_____

_____

_____

_____

_____

_____

_____

_____

_____

_____

 HEALTH TIP: Red cabbage is more nutrient dense than green cabbage, so go ahead and invite the red heads to dinner.

Daily Journal

DAY 22

FOOD

BREAKFAST TIME

Protein_____

Fat_____

Veggies_____

Low GI Carb_____

SNACK TIME

Protein_____

Fat_____

Veggies_____

Low GI Carb_____

LUNCH TIME

Protein_____

Fat_____

Veggies_____

Low GI Carb_____

SNACK TIME

Protein_____

Fat_____

Veggies_____

Low GI Carb_____

DINNERTIME

Protein_____

Fat_____

Veggies_____

Low GI Carb_____

WATER

☐ ☐ ☐ ☐
☐ ☐ ☐ ☐

EXERCISE

Cardio_____

Strength_____

HOW DO YOU FEEL?

_____
_____
_____
_____
_____
_____
_____
_____
_____
_____
_____
_____
_____
_____
_____

AFFIRMATION: Today is going to be a great day.

Daily Journal

DAY 23

FOOD

BREAKFAST TIME

Protein_____

Fat_____

Veggies_____

Low GI Carb_____

SNACK TIME

Protein_____

Fat_____

Veggies_____

Low GI Carb_____

LUNCH TIME

Protein_____

Fat_____

Veggies_____

Low GI Carb_____

SNACK TIME

Protein_____

Fat_____

Veggies_____

Low GI Carb_____

DINNERTIME

Protein_____

Fat_____

Veggies_____

Low GI Carb_____

WATER

☐ ☐ ☐ ☐
☐ ☐ ☐ ☐

EXERCISE

Cardio_____

Strength_____

HOW DO YOU FEEL?

_____

_____

_____

_____

_____

_____

_____

_____

_____

_____

_____

_____

_____

_____

_____

QUOTE: Look to your health; if you got it, praise God, and value it next to a good conscience; for health is the second blessing that we mortals are capable of; a blessing that money cannot buy.
~IZAAK WALTON

Daily Journal

DAY 24

FOOD

BREAKFAST TIME

Protein_____

Fat_____

Veggies_____

Low GI Carb_____

SNACK TIME

Protein_____

Fat_____

Veggies_____

Low GI Carb_____

LUNCH TIME

Protein_____

Fat_____

Veggies_____

Low GI Carb_____

SNACK TIME

Protein_____

Fat_____

Veggies_____

Low GI Carb_____

DINNERTIME

Protein_____

Fat_____

Veggies_____

Low GI Carb_____

WATER

☐ ☐ ☐ ☐
☐ ☐ ☐ ☐

EXERCISE

Cardio_____

Strength_____

HOW DO YOU FEEL?

_____
_____
_____
_____
_____
_____
_____
_____
_____
_____
_____
_____
_____
_____
_____

HEALTH TIP: Be kind to yourself. This process is about breaking bad habits and creating new ones, one habit at a time. It's not about doing anything perfectly. Do your best and you will see results.

Daily Journal

DAY 25

FOOD

BREAKFAST TIME

Protein_____

Fat_____

Veggies_____

Low GI Carb_____

SNACK TIME

Protein_____

Fat_____

Veggies_____

Low GI Carb_____

LUNCH TIME

Protein_____

Fat_____

Veggies_____

Low GI Carb_____

SNACK TIME

Protein_____

Fat_____

Veggies_____

Low GI Carb_____

DINNERTIME

Protein_____

Fat_____

Veggies_____

Low GI Carb_____

WATER

☐ ☐ ☐ ☐
☐ ☐ ☐ ☐

EXERCISE

Cardio_____

Strength_____

HOW DO YOU FEEL?

_____

_____

_____

_____

_____

_____

_____

_____

_____

_____

_____

_____

_____

_____

_____

_____

 AFFIRMATION: I have the strength to carry me through.

Daily Journal

DAY 26

FOOD

BREAKFAST TIME

Protein_____

Fat_____

Veggies_____

Low GI Carb_____

SNACK TIME

Protein_____

Fat_____

Veggies_____

Low GI Carb_____

LUNCH TIME

Protein_____

Fat_____

Veggies_____

Low GI Carb_____

SNACK TIME

Protein_____

Fat_____

Veggies_____

Low GI Carb_____

DINNERTIME

Protein_____

Fat_____

Veggies_____

Low GI Carb_____

WATER

☐ ☐ ☐ ☐
☐ ☐ ☐ ☐

EXERCISE

Cardio_____

Strength_____

HOW DO YOU FEEL?

_____
_____
_____
_____
_____
_____
_____
_____
_____
_____
_____
_____
_____
_____
_____

QUOTE: Most people have no idea of the giant capacity we can immediately command when we focus all our resources on mastering a single area of our lives.

~TONY ROBBINS

Daily Journal

DAY 27

FOOD

BREAKFAST TIME

Protein_____

Fat_____

Veggies_____

Low GI Carb_____

SNACK TIME

Protein_____

Fat_____

Veggies_____

Low GI Carb_____

LUNCH TIME

Protein_____

Fat_____

Veggies_____

Low GI Carb_____

SNACK TIME

Protein_____

Fat_____

Veggies_____

Low GI Carb_____

DINNERTIME

Protein_____

Fat_____

Veggies_____

Low GI Carb_____

WATER

☐ ☐ ☐ ☐
☐ ☐ ☐ ☐

EXERCISE

Cardio_____

Strength_____

HOW DO YOU FEEL?

_____

_____

_____

_____

_____

_____

_____

_____

_____

_____

_____

_____

_____

_____

_____

 HEALTH TIP: Taking a hot shower can have a blood glucose lowering affect.

Daily Journal

DAY 28

FOOD

BREAKFAST TIME

Protein_____

Fat_____

Veggies_____

Low GI Carb_____

SNACK TIME

Protein_____

Fat_____

Veggies_____

Low GI Carb_____

LUNCH TIME

Protein_____

Fat_____

Veggies_____

Low GI Carb_____

SNACK TIME

Protein_____

Fat_____

Veggies_____

Low GI Carb_____

DINNERTIME

Protein_____

Fat_____

Veggies_____

Low GI Carb_____

WATER

☐ ☐ ☐ ☐
☐ ☐ ☐ ☐

EXERCISE

Cardio_____

Strength_____

HOW DO YOU FEEL?

_____
_____
_____
_____
_____
_____
_____
_____
_____
_____
_____
_____
_____
_____

AFFIRMATION: I am proud of myself.

Daily Journal

DAY 29

FOOD

BREAKFAST TIME

Protein_____

Fat_____

Veggies_____

Low GI Carb_____

SNACK TIME

Protein_____

Fat_____

Veggies_____

Low GI Carb_____

LUNCH TIME

Protein_____

Fat_____

Veggies_____

Low GI Carb_____

SNACK TIME

Protein_____

Fat_____

Veggies_____

Low GI Carb_____

DINNERTIME

Protein_____

Fat_____

Veggies_____

Low GI Carb_____

WATER

☐ ☐ ☐ ☐
☐ ☐ ☐ ☐

EXERCISE

Cardio_____

Strength_____

HOW DO YOU FEEL?

_____
_____
_____
_____
_____
_____
_____
_____
_____
_____
_____
_____
_____
_____
_____
_____

HEALTH TIP: During exercise, raising your hands above your heart will increase intensity. If things are too intense, lower your arms back down.

Daily Journal

DAY 30

FOOD

BREAKFAST TIME

Protein_____

Fat_____

Veggies_____

Low GI Carb_____

SNACK TIME

Protein_____

Fat_____

Veggies_____

Low GI Carb_____

LUNCH TIME

Protein_____

Fat_____

Veggies_____

Low GI Carb_____

SNACK TIME

Protein_____

Fat_____

Veggies_____

Low GI Carb_____

DINNERTIME

Protein_____

Fat_____

Veggies_____

Low GI Carb_____

WATER

☐ ☐ ☐ ☐
☐ ☐ ☐ ☐

EXERCISE

Cardio_____

Strength_____

HOW DO YOU FEEL?

_____

_____

_____

_____

_____

_____

_____

_____

_____

_____

_____

_____

_____

_____

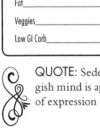

QUOTE: Sedentary people are apt to have sluggish minds. A sluggish mind is apt to be reflected in flabbiness of a body and dullness of expression that invites no interest and gets none.

~ROSE FITZGERALD KENNEDY

Daily Journal

DAY 31

FOOD

BREAKFAST TIME

Protein_____

Fat_____

Veggies_____

Low GI Carb_____

SNACK TIME

Protein_____

Fat_____

Veggies_____

Low GI Carb_____

LUNCH TIME

Protein_____

Fat_____

Veggies_____

Low GI Carb_____

SNACK TIME

Protein_____

Fat_____

Veggies_____

Low GI Carb_____

DINNERTIME

Protein_____

Fat_____

Veggies_____

Low GI Carb_____

WATER

☐ ☐ ☐ ☐
☐ ☐ ☐ ☐

EXERCISE

Cardio_____

Strength_____

HOW DO YOU FEEL?

_____
_____
_____
_____
_____
_____
_____
_____
_____
_____
_____
_____
_____
_____

AFFIRMATION: I visualize my future and the brightness is stunning.

Daily Journal
DAY 32

FOOD

BREAKFAST TIME

Protein_____

Fat_____

Veggies_____

Low GI Carb_____

SNACK TIME

Protein_____

Fat_____

Veggies_____

Low GI Carb_____

LUNCH TIME

Protein_____

Fat_____

Veggies_____

Low GI Carb_____

SNACK TIME

Protein_____

Fat_____

Veggies_____

Low GI Carb_____

DINNERTIME

Protein_____

Fat_____

Veggies_____

Low GI Carb_____

WATER

☐ ☐ ☐ ☐
☐ ☐ ☐ ☐

EXERCISE

Cardio_____

Strength_____

HOW DO
YOU FEEL?

_____
_____
_____
_____
_____
_____
_____
_____
_____
_____
_____
_____
_____
_____
_____

 QUOTE: If I had not already been meditating, I would certainly have to start. I've treated my own depression for many years with exercise and meditation and I've found that to be tremendous help.
~JUDY COLLINS

Daily Journal

DAY 33

FOOD

BREAKFAST TIME

Protein_____

Fat_____

Veggies_____

Low GI Carb_____

SNACK TIME

Protein_____

Fat_____

Veggies_____

Low GI Carb_____

LUNCH TIME

Protein_____

Fat_____

Veggies_____

Low GI Carb_____

SNACK TIME

Protein_____

Fat_____

Veggies_____

Low GI Carb_____

DINNERTIME

Protein_____

Fat_____

Veggies_____

Low GI Carb_____

WATER

☐ ☐ ☐ ☐
☐ ☐ ☐ ☐

EXERCISE

Cardio_____

Strength_____

HOW DO YOU FEEL?

_____

_____

_____

_____

_____

_____

_____

_____

_____

_____

_____

_____

_____

_____

_____

HEALTH TIP: Don't drink your fruit, eat it. Fruit juice is nutritious, but all the fiber is removed so it becomes high glycemic. Apples, berries, and oranges are low glycemic when eaten whole. The only exception to this rule is pineapple juice. Just don't exceed 4 oz. at a time.

Daily Journal

DAY 34

FOOD

BREAKFAST TIME

Protein_____

Fat_____

Veggies_____

Low GI Carb_____

SNACK TIME

Protein_____

Fat_____

Veggies_____

Low GI Carb_____

LUNCH TIME

Protein_____

Fat_____

Veggies_____

Low GI Carb_____

SNACK TIME

Protein_____

Fat_____

Veggies_____

Low GI Carb_____

DINNERTIME

Protein_____

Fat_____

Veggies_____

Low GI Carb_____

WATER

☐ ☐ ☐ ☐
☐ ☐ ☐ ☐

EXERCISE

Cardio_____

Strength_____

HOW DO YOU FEEL?

_____
_____
_____
_____
_____
_____
_____
_____
_____
_____
_____
_____
_____
_____

AFFIRMATION: At last at last, the past is past; I've broken free and won. Now it's time to love myself and really have some fun.

Daily Journal

DAY 35

FOOD

BREAKFAST TIME

Protein_____

Fat_____

Veggies_____

Low GI Carb_____

SNACK TIME

Protein_____

Fat_____

Veggies_____

Low GI Carb_____

LUNCH TIME

Protein_____

Fat_____

Veggies_____

Low GI Carb_____

SNACK TIME

Protein_____

Fat_____

Veggies_____

Low GI Carb_____

DINNERTIME

Protein_____

Fat_____

Veggies_____

Low GI Carb_____

WATER

☐ ☐ ☐ ☐
☐ ☐ ☐ ☐

EXERCISE

Cardio_____

Strength_____

HOW DO YOU FEEL?

_____
_____
_____
_____
_____
_____
_____
_____
_____
_____
_____
_____
_____
_____
_____
_____

QUOTE: For changes to be of any true value, they've got to be lasting and consistent.

~TONY ROBBINS

Daily Journal

DAY 36

FOOD

BREAKFAST TIME

Protein_____

Fat_____

Veggies_____

Low GI Carb_____

SNACK TIME

Protein_____

Fat_____

Veggies_____

Low GI Carb_____

LUNCH TIME

Protein_____

Fat_____

Veggies_____

Low GI Carb_____

SNACK TIME

Protein_____

Fat_____

Veggies_____

Low GI Carb_____

DINNERTIME

Protein_____

Fat_____

Veggies_____

Low GI Carb_____

WATER

☐ ☐ ☐ ☐
☐ ☐ ☐ ☐

EXERCISE

Cardio_____

Strength_____

HOW DO YOU FEEL?

_____

_____

_____

_____

_____

_____

_____

_____

_____

_____

_____

_____

_____

_____

_____

_____

 TO DO: Measure today . . .

Daily Journal

DAY 37

FOOD

BREAKFAST TIME

Protein_____

Fat_____

Veggies_____

Low GI Carb_____

SNACK TIME

Protein_____

Fat_____

Veggies_____

Low GI Carb_____

LUNCH TIME

Protein_____

Fat_____

Veggies_____

Low GI Carb_____

SNACK TIME

Protein_____

Fat_____

Veggies_____

Low GI Carb_____

DINNERTIME

Protein_____

Fat_____

Veggies_____

Low GI Carb_____

WATER

☐ ☐ ☐ ☐
☐ ☐ ☐ ☐

EXERCISE

Cardio_____

Strength_____

HOW DO YOU FEEL?

_____

_____

_____

_____

_____

_____

_____

_____

_____

_____

_____

_____

_____

_____

HEALTH TIP: Choose yams instead of potatoes for a lower GI carb.

Daily Journal

DAY 38

FOOD

BREAKFAST TIME

Protein_____

Fat_____

Veggies_____

Low GI Carb_____

SNACK TIME

Protein_____

Fat_____

Veggies_____

Low GI Carb_____

LUNCH TIME

Protein_____

Fat_____

Veggies_____

Low GI Carb_____

SNACK TIME

Protein_____

Fat_____

Veggies_____

Low GI Carb_____

DINNERTIME

Protein_____

Fat_____

Veggies_____

Low GI Carb_____

WATER

☐ ☐ ☐ ☐
☐ ☐ ☐ ☐

EXERCISE

Cardio_____

Strength_____

HOW DO YOU FEEL?

_____
_____
_____
_____
_____
_____
_____
_____
_____
_____
_____
_____
_____
_____
_____

QUOTE: To me, good health is more than just exercise and diet. It's really a point of view and a mental attitude you have about yourself.

~ANGELA LANSBURY

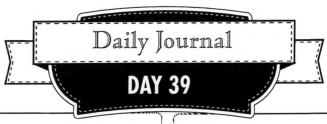

Daily Journal

DAY 39

FOOD

BREAKFAST TIME

Protein_____

Fat_____

Veggies_____

Low GI Carb_____

SNACK TIME

Protein_____

Fat_____

Veggies_____

Low GI Carb_____

LUNCH TIME

Protein_____

Fat_____

Veggies_____

Low GI Carb_____

SNACK TIME

Protein_____

Fat_____

Veggies_____

Low GI Carb_____

DINNERTIME

Protein_____

Fat_____

Veggies_____

Low GI Carb_____

WATER

☐ ☐ ☐ ☐
☐ ☐ ☐ ☐

EXERCISE

Cardio_____

Strength_____

HOW DO YOU FEEL?

_____
_____
_____
_____
_____
_____
_____
_____
_____
_____
_____
_____
_____
_____
_____
_____

AFFIRMATION: I love to exercise.

Daily Journal
DAY 40

FOOD

BREAKFAST TIME

Protein_____

Fat_____

Veggies_____

Low GI Carb_____

SNACK TIME

Protein_____

Fat_____

Veggies_____

Low GI Carb_____

LUNCH TIME

Protein_____

Fat_____

Veggies_____

Low GI Carb_____

SNACK TIME

Protein_____

Fat_____

Veggies_____

Low GI Carb_____

DINNERTIME

Protein_____

Fat_____

Veggies_____

Low GI Carb_____

WATER

☐ ☐ ☐ ☐
☐ ☐ ☐ ☐

EXERCISE

Cardio_____

Strength_____

HOW DO YOU FEEL?

_____
_____
_____
_____
_____
_____
_____
_____
_____
_____
_____
_____
_____
_____
_____

 HEALTH TIP: When doing lunges or squats, don't let your knee pass your toes. Look in the mirror, so when you come down, you can make sure you line up your knee above your ankle.

Daily Journal

DAY 41

FOOD

BREAKFAST TIME

Protein_____

Fat_____

Veggies_____

Low GI Carb_____

SNACK TIME

Protein_____

Fat_____

Veggies_____

Low GI Carb_____

LUNCH TIME

Protein_____

Fat_____

Veggies_____

Low GI Carb_____

SNACK TIME

Protein_____

Fat_____

Veggies_____

Low GI Carb_____

DINNERTIME

Protein_____

Fat_____

Veggies_____

Low GI Carb_____

WATER

☐ ☐ ☐ ☐
☐ ☐ ☐ ☐

EXERCISE

Cardio_____

Strength_____

HOW DO YOU FEEL?

_____
_____
_____
_____
_____
_____
_____
_____
_____
_____
_____
_____
_____
_____
_____
_____

QUOTE: It matters more what's in a women's face, than what's on it.

~CLAUDETTE COLBERT

Daily Journal

DAY 42

FOOD

BREAKFAST TIME

Protein_____

Fat_____

Veggies_____

Low GI Carb_____

SNACK TIME

Protein_____

Fat_____

Veggies_____

Low GI Carb_____

LUNCH TIME

Protein_____

Fat_____

Veggies_____

Low GI Carb_____

SNACK TIME

Protein_____

Fat_____

Veggies_____

Low GI Carb_____

DINNERTIME

Protein_____

Fat_____

Veggies_____

Low GI Carb_____

WATER

☐ ☐ ☐ ☐
☐ ☐ ☐ ☐

EXERCISE

Cardio_____

Strength_____

HOW DO YOU FEEL?

_____
_____
_____
_____
_____
_____
_____
_____
_____
_____
_____
_____
_____
_____

AFFIRMATION: I will make healthy choices all day.

Daily Journal

DAY 43

FOOD

BREAKFAST TIME

Protein_____

Fat_____

Veggies_____

Low GI Carb_____

SNACK TIME

Protein_____

Fat_____

Veggies_____

Low GI Carb_____

LUNCH TIME

Protein_____

Fat_____

Veggies_____

Low GI Carb_____

SNACK TIME

Protein_____

Fat_____

Veggies_____

Low GI Carb_____

DINNERTIME

Protein_____

Fat_____

Veggies_____

Low GI Carb_____

WATER

☐ ☐ ☐ ☐
☐ ☐ ☐ ☐

EXERCISE

Cardio_____

Strength_____

HOW DO YOU FEEL?

_____
_____
_____
_____
_____
_____
_____
_____
_____
_____
_____
_____
_____
_____

QUOTE: To accomplish great things, we must not only act, but also dream; not only plan, but also believe.

~ANATOLE FRANCE

Daily Journal

DAY 44

FOOD

BREAKFAST TIME

Protein_____

Fat_____

Veggies_____

Low GI Carb_____

SNACK TIME

Protein_____

Fat_____

Veggies_____

Low GI Carb_____

LUNCH TIME

Protein_____

Fat_____

Veggies_____

Low GI Carb_____

SNACK TIME

Protein_____

Fat_____

Veggies_____

Low GI Carb_____

DINNERTIME

Protein_____

Fat_____

Veggies_____

Low GI Carb_____

WATER

☐ ☐ ☐ ☐
☐ ☐ ☐ ☐

EXERCISE

Cardio_____

Strength_____

HOW DO YOU FEEL?

_____
_____
_____
_____
_____
_____
_____
_____
_____
_____
_____
_____
_____
_____

HEALTH TIP: Adding turmeric to your food has many health benefits. In addition to aiding in weight loss, it is also a natural liver detoxifier, prevents certain cancers, and it's an anti-inflammatory, which can really help with sore joints and arthritis.

Daily Journal
DAY 45

FOOD

BREAKFAST TIME

Protein_____

Fat_____

Veggies_____

Low GI Carb_____

SNACK TIME

Protein_____

Fat_____

Veggies_____

Low GI Carb_____

LUNCH TIME

Protein_____

Fat_____

Veggies_____

Low GI Carb_____

SNACK TIME

Protein_____

Fat_____

Veggies_____

Low GI Carb_____

DINNERTIME

Protein_____

Fat_____

Veggies_____

Low GI Carb_____

WATER

☐ ☐ ☐ ☐
☐ ☐ ☐ ☐

EXERCISE

Cardio_____

Strength_____

HOW DO YOU FEEL?

_____
_____
_____
_____
_____
_____
_____
_____
_____
_____
_____
_____
_____
_____
_____
_____

AFFIRMATION: All the joy I need is within me now.

Daily Journal

DAY 46

FOOD

BREAKFAST TIME

Protein_____

Fat_____

Veggies_____

Low GI Carb_____

SNACK TIME

Protein_____

Fat_____

Veggies_____

Low GI Carb_____

LUNCH TIME

Protein_____

Fat_____

Veggies_____

Low GI Carb_____

SNACK TIME

Protein_____

Fat_____

Veggies_____

Low GI Carb_____

DINNERTIME

Protein_____

Fat_____

Veggies_____

Low GI Carb_____

WATER

☐ ☐ ☐ ☐
☐ ☐ ☐ ☐

EXERCISE

Cardio_____

Strength_____

HOW DO YOU FEEL?

_____
_____
_____
_____
_____
_____
_____
_____
_____
_____
_____
_____
_____
_____

AFFIRMATION: I am accomplishing my goals.

Daily Journal

DAY 47

FOOD

BREAKFAST TIME

Protein_____

Fat_____

Veggies_____

Low GI Carb_____

SNACK TIME

Protein_____

Fat_____

Veggies_____

Low GI Carb_____

LUNCH TIME

Protein_____

Fat_____

Veggies_____

Low GI Carb_____

SNACK TIME

Protein_____

Fat_____

Veggies_____

Low GI Carb_____

DINNERTIME

Protein_____

Fat_____

Veggies_____

Low GI Carb_____

WATER

☐ ☐ ☐ ☐
☐ ☐ ☐ ☐

EXERCISE

Cardio_____

Strength_____

HOW DO YOU FEEL?

_____
_____
_____
_____
_____
_____
_____
_____
_____
_____
_____
_____
_____
_____
_____
_____
_____

HEALTH TIP: Eat your carbs, even low GI ones last. Starting your meal with one serving of healthy fat and some protein will lower the GI impact of the whole meal, keeping you in a fat burning zone.

Daily Journal

DAY 48

FOOD

BREAKFAST TIME

Protein_____

Fat_____

Veggies_____

Low GI Carb_____

SNACK TIME

Protein_____

Fat_____

Veggies_____

Low GI Carb_____

LUNCH TIME

Protein_____

Fat_____

Veggies_____

Low GI Carb_____

SNACK TIME

Protein_____

Fat_____

Veggies_____

Low GI Carb_____

DINNERTIME

Protein_____

Fat_____

Veggies_____

Low GI Carb_____

WATER

☐ ☐ ☐ ☐
☐ ☐ ☐ ☐

EXERCISE

Cardio_____

Strength_____

HOW DO YOU FEEL?

_____

_____

_____

_____

_____

_____

_____

_____

_____

_____

_____

_____

_____

_____

_____

QUOTE: Nothing happens unless we first dream.

~CARL SANDBURG

Daily Journal

DAY 49

FOOD

BREAKFAST TIME

Protein_____

Fat_____

Veggies_____

Low GI Carb_____

SNACK TIME

Protein_____

Fat_____

Veggies_____

Low GI Carb_____

LUNCH TIME

Protein_____

Fat_____

Veggies_____

Low GI Carb_____

SNACK TIME

Protein_____

Fat_____

Veggies_____

Low GI Carb_____

DINNERTIME

Protein_____

Fat_____

Veggies_____

Low GI Carb_____

WATER

☐ ☐ ☐ ☐
☐ ☐ ☐ ☐

EXERCISE

Cardio_____

Strength_____

HOW DO YOU FEEL?

_____

_____

_____

_____

_____

_____

_____

_____

_____

_____

_____

_____

_____

_____

 HEALTH TIP: Focus equals reality. Focus on the results you want, not how hard or how long a process it is. Keep your mind's eye on the prize!

Daily Journal

DAY 50

FOOD

BREAKFAST TIME

Protein_____

Fat_____

Veggies_____

Low GI Carb_____

SNACK TIME

Protein_____

Fat_____

Veggies_____

Low GI Carb_____

LUNCH TIME

Protein_____

Fat_____

Veggies_____

Low GI Carb_____

SNACK TIME

Protein_____

Fat_____

Veggies_____

Low GI Carb_____

DINNERTIME

Protein_____

Fat_____

Veggies_____

Low GI Carb_____

WATER

☐ ☐ ☐ ☐
☐ ☐ ☐ ☐

EXERCISE

Cardio_____

Strength_____

HOW DO YOU FEEL?

_____
_____
_____
_____
_____
_____
_____
_____
_____
_____
_____
_____
_____
_____
_____

QUOTE: Any time you sincerely want to make a change, the first thing you must do is to raise your standards. When people ask me what really changed my life eight years ago, I tell them that absolutely the most important thing was changing what I demanded of myself. I wrote down all the things I would no longer accept in my life, all the things I would no longer tolerate, and all the things that I aspired to becoming.

~ANTHONY ROBBINS

Daily Journal

DAY 51

FOOD

BREAKFAST TIME

Protein_____

Fat_____

Veggies_____

Low GI Carb_____

SNACK TIME

Protein_____

Fat_____

Veggies_____

Low GI Carb_____

LUNCH TIME

Protein_____

Fat_____

Veggies_____

Low GI Carb_____

SNACK TIME

Protein_____

Fat_____

Veggies_____

Low GI Carb_____

DINNERTIME

Protein_____

Fat_____

Veggies_____

Low GI Carb_____

WATER

☐ ☐ ☐ ☐
☐ ☐ ☐ ☐

EXERCISE

Cardio_____

Strength_____

HOW DO YOU FEEL?

_____

_____

_____

_____

_____

_____

_____

_____

_____

_____

_____

_____

_____

_____

 HEALTH TIP: If five minutes of cardio is all you can do then great! Do five minutes. Try adding five minutes later in the same day and you have done 10 minutes of cardio in a single day. You can add on a minute or two from there.

Daily Journal

DAY 52

FOOD

BREAKFAST TIME

Protein_____

Fat_____

Veggies_____

Low GI Carb_____

SNACK TIME

Protein_____

Fat_____

Veggies_____

Low GI Carb_____

LUNCH TIME

Protein_____

Fat_____

Veggies_____

Low GI Carb_____

SNACK TIME

Protein_____

Fat_____

Veggies_____

Low GI Carb_____

DINNERTIME

Protein_____

Fat_____

Veggies_____

Low GI Carb_____

WATER

☐ ☐ ☐ ☐
☐ ☐ ☐ ☐

EXERCISE

Cardio_____

Strength_____

HOW DO YOU FEEL?

_____
_____
_____
_____
_____
_____
_____
_____
_____
_____
_____
_____
_____
_____

AFFIRMATION: Every day, in every way, I'm feeling stronger and stronger.

Daily Journal

DAY 53

FOOD

BREAKFAST TIME

Protein_____

Fat_____

Veggies_____

Low GI Carb_____

SNACK TIME

Protein_____

Fat_____

Veggies_____

Low GI Carb_____

LUNCH TIME

Protein_____

Fat_____

Veggies_____

Low GI Carb_____

SNACK TIME

Protein_____

Fat_____

Veggies_____

Low GI Carb_____

DINNERTIME

Protein_____

Fat_____

Veggies_____

Low GI Carb_____

WATER

☐ ☐ ☐ ☐
☐ ☐ ☐ ☐

EXERCISE

Cardio_____

Strength_____

HOW DO YOU FEEL?

_____
_____
_____
_____
_____
_____
_____
_____
_____
_____
_____
_____
_____
_____
_____
_____

HEALTH TIP: Go for original oatmeal. The instant kind is processed and high glycemic.

Daily Journal

DAY 54

FOOD

BREAKFAST TIME

Protein_____

Fat_____

Veggies_____

Low GI Carb_____

SNACK TIME

Protein_____

Fat_____

Veggies_____

Low GI Carb_____

LUNCH TIME

Protein_____

Fat_____

Veggies_____

Low GI Carb_____

SNACK TIME

Protein_____

Fat_____

Veggies_____

Low GI Carb_____

DINNERTIME

Protein_____

Fat_____

Veggies_____

Low GI Carb_____

WATER

☐ ☐ ☐ ☐
☐ ☐ ☐ ☐

EXERCISE

Cardio_____

Strength_____

HOW DO YOU FEEL?

_____
_____
_____
_____
_____
_____
_____
_____
_____
_____
_____
_____
_____
_____

QUOTE: It isn't where you come from; it's where you're going that counts.

~ELLA FITZGERALD

Daily Journal

DAY 55

FOOD

BREAKFAST TIME

Protein_____

Fat_____

Veggies_____

Low GI Carb_____

SNACK TIME

Protein_____

Fat_____

Veggies_____

Low GI Carb_____

LUNCH TIME

Protein_____

Fat_____

Veggies_____

Low GI Carb_____

SNACK TIME

Protein_____

Fat_____

Veggies_____

Low GI Carb_____

DINNERTIME

Protein_____

Fat_____

Veggies_____

Low GI Carb_____

WATER

☐ ☐ ☐ ☐
☐ ☐ ☐ ☐

EXERCISE

Cardio_____

Strength_____

HOW DO YOU FEEL?

_____
_____
_____
_____
_____
_____
_____
_____
_____
_____
_____
_____
_____
_____
_____

 AFFIRMATION: Faith is the fuel that fires success.

Daily Journal

DAY 56

FOOD

BREAKFAST TIME

Protein_____

Fat_____

Veggies_____

Low GI Carb_____

SNACK TIME

Protein_____

Fat_____

Veggies_____

Low GI Carb_____

LUNCH TIME

Protein_____

Fat_____

Veggies_____

Low GI Carb_____

SNACK TIME

Protein_____

Fat_____

Veggies_____

Low GI Carb_____

DINNERTIME

Protein_____

Fat_____

Veggies_____

Low GI Carb_____

WATER

☐ ☐ ☐ ☐
☐ ☐ ☐ ☐

EXERCISE

Cardio_____

Strength_____

HOW DO YOU FEEL?

_____

_____

_____

_____

_____

_____

_____

_____

_____

_____

_____

_____

_____

_____

_____

QUOTE: A real decision is measured by the fact that you've taken a new action. If there is no action then you truly haven't decided.
~TONY ROBBINS

Daily Journal

DAY 57

FOOD

BREAKFAST TIME

Protein_____

Fat_____

Veggies_____

Low GI Carb_____

SNACK TIME

Protein_____

Fat_____

Veggies_____

Low GI Carb_____

LUNCH TIME

Protein_____

Fat_____

Veggies_____

Low GI Carb_____

SNACK TIME

Protein_____

Fat_____

Veggies_____

Low GI Carb_____

DINNERTIME

Protein_____

Fat_____

Veggies_____

Low GI Carb_____

WATER

☐ ☐ ☐ ☐
☐ ☐ ☐ ☐

EXERCISE

Cardio_____

Strength_____

HOW DO YOU FEEL?

_____
_____
_____
_____
_____
_____
_____
_____
_____
_____
_____
_____
_____
_____
_____

TO DO: Measure today . . .

Daily Journal

DAY 58

FOOD

BREAKFAST TIME

Protein_____

Fat_____

Veggies_____

Low GI Carb_____

SNACK TIME

Protein_____

Fat_____

Veggies_____

Low GI Carb_____

LUNCH TIME

Protein_____

Fat_____

Veggies_____

Low GI Carb_____

SNACK TIME

Protein_____

Fat_____

Veggies_____

Low GI Carb_____

DINNERTIME

Protein_____

Fat_____

Veggies_____

Low GI Carb_____

WATER

☐ ☐ ☐ ☐
☐ ☐ ☐ ☐

EXERCISE

Cardio_____

Strength_____

HOW DO YOU FEEL?

_____
_____
_____
_____
_____
_____
_____
_____
_____
_____
_____
_____
_____
_____

HEALTH TIP: Have your fruits and veggies pre cut or peeled for the next day or so. It makes it so much easier to make your best choice in a hurry.

FOOD

BREAKFAST TIME

Protein_____

Fat_____

Veggies_____

Low GI Carb_____

SNACK TIME

Protein_____

Fat_____

Veggies_____

Low GI Carb_____

LUNCH TIME

Protein_____

Fat_____

Veggies_____

Low GI Carb_____

SNACK TIME

Protein_____

Fat_____

Veggies_____

Low GI Carb_____

DINNERTIME

Protein_____

Fat_____

Veggies_____

Low GI Carb_____

WATER

☐ ☐ ☐ ☐
☐ ☐ ☐ ☐

EXERCISE

Cardio_____

Strength_____

HOW DO YOU FEEL?

_____

_____

_____

_____

_____

_____

_____

_____

_____

_____

_____

_____

_____

_____

AFFIRMATION: At last at last, the past is past I've broken free and won. Now it's time to love myself and really have some fun.

Daily Journal

DAY 60

FOOD

BREAKFAST TIME

Protein_____

Fat_____

Veggies_____

Low GI Carb_____

SNACK TIME

Protein_____

Fat_____

Veggies_____

Low GI Carb_____

LUNCH TIME

Protein_____

Fat_____

Veggies_____

Low GI Carb_____

SNACK TIME

Protein_____

Fat_____

Veggies_____

Low GI Carb_____

DINNERTIME

Protein_____

Fat_____

Veggies_____

Low GI Carb_____

WATER

☐ ☐ ☐ ☐
☐ ☐ ☐ ☐

EXERCISE

Cardio_____

Strength_____

HOW DO YOU FEEL?

_____
_____
_____
_____
_____
_____
_____
_____
_____
_____
_____
_____
_____
_____
_____
_____

QUOTE: I know the price of success: dedication, hard work, and an unremitting devotion to the things that you want to see happen.

~FRANK LLOYD WRIGHT

Daily Journal

DAY 61

FOOD

BREAKFAST TIME

Protein_____

Fat_____

Veggies_____

Low GI Carb_____

SNACK TIME

Protein_____

Fat_____

Veggies_____

Low GI Carb_____

LUNCH TIME

Protein_____

Fat_____

Veggies_____

Low GI Carb_____

SNACK TIME

Protein_____

Fat_____

Veggies_____

Low GI Carb_____

DINNERTIME

Protein_____

Fat_____

Veggies_____

Low GI Carb_____

WATER

☐ ☐ ☐ ☐
☐ ☐ ☐ ☐

EXERCISE

Cardio_____

Strength_____

HOW DO YOU FEEL?

_____

_____

_____

_____

_____

_____

_____

_____

_____

_____

_____

_____

_____

_____

 AFFIRMATION: I visualize my future and the brightness is stunning.

Daily Journal

DAY 62

FOOD

BREAKFAST TIME

Protein_____

Fat_____

Veggies_____

Low GI Carb_____

SNACK TIME

Protein_____

Fat_____

Veggies_____

Low GI Carb_____

LUNCH TIME

Protein_____

Fat_____

Veggies_____

Low GI Carb_____

SNACK TIME

Protein_____

Fat_____

Veggies_____

Low GI Carb_____

DINNERTIME

Protein_____

Fat_____

Veggies_____

Low GI Carb_____

WATER

☐ ☐ ☐ ☐
☐ ☐ ☐ ☐

EXERCISE

Cardio_____

Strength_____

HOW DO YOU FEEL?

_____
_____
_____
_____
_____
_____
_____
_____
_____
_____
_____
_____
_____
_____
_____

QUOTE: First say to yourself what you would be; then do what you have to do.

~EPICTETUS

Daily Journal

DAY 63

FOOD

BREAKFAST TIME

Protein_____

Fat_____

Veggies_____

Low GI Carb_____

SNACK TIME

Protein_____

Fat_____

Veggies_____

Low GI Carb_____

LUNCH TIME

Protein_____

Fat_____

Veggies_____

Low GI Carb_____

SNACK TIME

Protein_____

Fat_____

Veggies_____

Low GI Carb_____

DINNERTIME

Protein_____

Fat_____

Veggies_____

Low GI Carb_____

WATER

☐ ☐ ☐ ☐
☐ ☐ ☐ ☐

EXERCISE

Cardio_____

Strength_____

HOW DO YOU FEEL?

_____
_____
_____
_____
_____
_____
_____
_____
_____
_____
_____
_____
_____
_____
_____
_____
_____
_____

 HEALTH TIP: Alcohol reduces glucose released by the liver which can result in low blood sugar levels, which can lead to overeating. Remember you don't want your blood sugars too high, or too low.

Daily Journal

DAY 64

FOOD

BREAKFAST TIME

Protein_____

Fat_____

Veggies_____

Low GI Carb_____

SNACK TIME

Protein_____

Fat_____

Veggies_____

Low GI Carb_____

LUNCH TIME

Protein_____

Fat_____

Veggies_____

Low GI Carb_____

SNACK TIME

Protein_____

Fat_____

Veggies_____

Low GI Carb_____

DINNERTIME

Protein_____

Fat_____

Veggies_____

Low GI Carb_____

WATER

☐ ☐ ☐ ☐
☐ ☐ ☐ ☐

EXERCISE

Cardio_____

Strength_____

HOW DO YOU FEEL?

_____

_____

_____

_____

_____

_____

_____

_____

_____

_____

_____

_____

_____

AFFIRMATION: I am proud of myself.

Daily Journal

DAY 65

FOOD

BREAKFAST TIME

Protein_____

Fat_____

Veggies_____

Low GI Carb_____

SNACK TIME

Protein_____

Fat_____

Veggies_____

Low GI Carb_____

LUNCH TIME

Protein_____

Fat_____

Veggies_____

Low GI Carb_____

SNACK TIME

Protein_____

Fat_____

Veggies_____

Low GI Carb_____

DINNERTIME

Protein_____

Fat_____

Veggies_____

Low GI Carb_____

WATER

☐ ☐ ☐ ☐
☐ ☐ ☐ ☐

EXERCISE

Cardio_____

Strength_____

HOW DO YOU FEEL?

_____
_____
_____
_____
_____
_____
_____
_____
_____
_____
_____
_____
_____
_____
_____

QUOTE: Thought is the sculptor who can create the person you want to be.

~HENRY DAVID THOREAU

Daily Journal

DAY 66

FOOD

BREAKFAST TIME

Protein_____

Fat_____

Veggies_____

Low GI Carb_____

SNACK TIME

Protein_____

Fat_____

Veggies_____

Low GI Carb_____

LUNCH TIME

Protein_____

Fat_____

Veggies_____

Low GI Carb_____

SNACK TIME

Protein_____

Fat_____

Veggies_____

Low GI Carb_____

DINNERTIME

Protein_____

Fat_____

Veggies_____

Low GI Carb_____

WATER

☐ ☐ ☐ ☐
☐ ☐ ☐ ☐

EXERCISE

Cardio_____

Strength_____

HOW DO YOU FEEL?

_____

_____

_____

_____

_____

_____

_____

_____

_____

_____

_____

_____

_____

_____

_____

_____

 HEALTH TIP: Adding vinegar, lemon juice, or cinnamon can help lower the glycemic impact of your meal.

Daily Journal

DAY 67

FOOD

BREAKFAST TIME

Protein_____

Fat_____

Veggies_____

Low GI Carb_____

SNACK TIME

Protein_____

Fat_____

Veggies_____

Low GI Carb_____

LUNCH TIME

Protein_____

Fat_____

Veggies_____

Low GI Carb_____

SNACK TIME

Protein_____

Fat_____

Veggies_____

Low GI Carb_____

DINNERTIME

Protein_____

Fat_____

Veggies_____

Low GI Carb_____

WATER

☐ ☐ ☐ ☐
☐ ☐ ☐ ☐

EXERCISE

Cardio_____

Strength_____

HOW DO YOU FEEL?

_____
_____
_____
_____
_____
_____
_____
_____
_____
_____
_____
_____
_____
_____
_____
_____

QUOTE: It's more important to know where you're going than to get there quickly. Do not mistake activity for achievement.

~MABLE NEWCOMBER

153

Daily Journal
DAY 68

FOOD

BREAKFAST TIME

Protein_____

Fat_____

Veggies_____

Low GI Carb_____

SNACK TIME

Protein_____

Fat_____

Veggies_____

Low GI Carb_____

LUNCH TIME

Protein_____

Fat_____

Veggies_____

Low GI Carb_____

SNACK TIME

Protein_____

Fat_____

Veggies_____

Low GI Carb_____

DINNERTIME

Protein_____

Fat_____

Veggies_____

Low GI Carb_____

WATER

☐ ☐ ☐ ☐
☐ ☐ ☐ ☐

EXERCISE

Cardio_____

Strength_____

HOW DO YOU FEEL?

_____
_____
_____
_____
_____
_____
_____
_____
_____
_____
_____
_____
_____
_____

AFFIRMATION: I have the strength to carry me through.

Daily Journal

DAY 69

FOOD

BREAKFAST TIME

Protein_____

Fat_____

Veggies_____

Low GI Carb_____

SNACK TIME

Protein_____

Fat_____

Veggies_____

Low GI Carb_____

LUNCH TIME

Protein_____

Fat_____

Veggies_____

Low GI Carb_____

SNACK TIME

Protein_____

Fat_____

Veggies_____

Low GI Carb_____

DINNERTIME

Protein_____

Fat_____

Veggies_____

Low GI Carb_____

WATER

☐ ☐ ☐ ☐
☐ ☐ ☐ ☐

EXERCISE

Cardio_____

Strength_____

HOW DO YOU FEEL?

_____

_____

_____

_____

_____

_____

_____

_____

_____

_____

_____

_____

_____

_____

_____

_____

 HEALTH TIP: Get your family involved in eating more veggies. Studies have shown the more kids are take part in planting and caring for a garden the more they are interested in eating the veggies.

Daily Journal

DAY 70

FOOD

BREAKFAST TIME

Protein_____

Fat_____

Veggies_____

Low GI Carb_____

SNACK TIME

Protein_____

Fat_____

Veggies_____

Low GI Carb_____

LUNCH TIME

Protein_____

Fat_____

Veggies_____

Low GI Carb_____

SNACK TIME

Protein_____

Fat_____

Veggies_____

Low GI Carb_____

DINNERTIME

Protein_____

Fat_____

Veggies_____

Low GI Carb_____

WATER

☐ ☐ ☐ ☐
☐ ☐ ☐ ☐

EXERCISE

Cardio_____

Strength_____

HOW DO YOU FEEL?

_____
_____
_____
_____
_____
_____
_____
_____
_____
_____
_____
_____
_____
_____

QUOTE: Strategic planning is worthless unless you have a strategic vision.

~JOHN NAISBITT

Daily Journal

DAY 71

FOOD

BREAKFAST TIME

Protein_____

Fat_____

Veggies_____

Low GI Carb_____

SNACK TIME

Protein_____

Fat_____

Veggies_____

Low GI Carb_____

LUNCH TIME

Protein_____

Fat_____

Veggies_____

Low GI Carb_____

SNACK TIME

Protein_____

Fat_____

Veggies_____

Low GI Carb_____

DINNERTIME

Protein_____

Fat_____

Veggies_____

Low GI Carb_____

WATER

☐ ☐ ☐ ☐
☐ ☐ ☐ ☐

EXERCISE

Cardio_____

Strength_____

HOW DO YOU FEEL?

_____
_____
_____
_____
_____
_____
_____
_____
_____
_____
_____
_____
_____
_____
_____

HEALTH TIP: Garlic is considered a super food. It can help improve heart health, cholesterol levels and an antioxidant. It is also an immune booster; in fact 2-3 cloves can prevent a cold.

Daily Journal

DAY 72

FOOD

BREAKFAST TIME

Protein_____

Fat_____

Veggies_____

Low GI Carb_____

SNACK TIME

Protein_____

Fat_____

Veggies_____

Low GI Carb_____

LUNCH TIME

Protein_____

Fat_____

Veggies_____

Low GI Carb_____

SNACK TIME

Protein_____

Fat_____

Veggies_____

Low GI Carb_____

DINNERTIME

Protein_____

Fat_____

Veggies_____

Low GI Carb_____

WATER

☐ ☐ ☐ ☐
☐ ☐ ☐ ☐

EXERCISE

Cardio_____

Strength_____

HOW DO YOU FEEL?

_____
_____
_____
_____
_____
_____
_____
_____
_____
_____
_____
_____
_____
_____
_____

AFFIRMATION: Today is going to be a great day.

Daily Journal

DAY 73

FOOD

BREAKFAST TIME

Protein_____

Fat_____

Veggies_____

Low GI Carb_____

SNACK TIME

Protein_____

Fat_____

Veggies_____

Low GI Carb_____

LUNCH TIME

Protein_____

Fat_____

Veggies_____

Low GI Carb_____

SNACK TIME

Protein_____

Fat_____

Veggies_____

Low GI Carb_____

DINNERTIME

Protein_____

Fat_____

Veggies_____

Low GI Carb_____

WATER

☐ ☐ ☐ ☐
☐ ☐ ☐ ☐

EXERCISE

Cardio_____

Strength_____

HOW DO YOU FEEL?

_____

_____

_____

_____

_____

_____

_____

_____

_____

_____

_____

_____

_____

_____

_____

QUOTE: Goals are not only absolutely necessary to motivate us, they are essential to really keep us alive.

~ROBERT H. SCHULLER

Daily Journal

DAY 74

FOOD

BREAKFAST TIME

Protein_____

Fat_____

Veggies_____

Low GI Carb_____

SNACK TIME

Protein_____

Fat_____

Veggies_____

Low GI Carb_____

LUNCH TIME

Protein_____

Fat_____

Veggies_____

Low GI Carb_____

SNACK TIME

Protein_____

Fat_____

Veggies_____

Low GI Carb_____

DINNERTIME

Protein_____

Fat_____

Veggies_____

Low GI Carb_____

WATER

☐ ☐ ☐ ☐
☐ ☐ ☐ ☐

EXERCISE

Cardio_____

Strength_____

HOW DO YOU FEEL?

_____
_____
_____
_____
_____
_____
_____
_____
_____
_____
_____
_____
_____
_____

HEALTH TIP: To raise your heart rate during resistance training, work two muscle groups at a time. For example, Lunges and bicep curls or squats with a front raise.

Daily Journal

DAY 75

FOOD

BREAKFAST TIME

Protein_____

Fat_____

Veggies_____

Low GI Carb_____

SNACK TIME

Protein_____

Fat_____

Veggies_____

Low GI Carb_____

LUNCH TIME

Protein_____

Fat_____

Veggies_____

Low GI Carb_____

SNACK TIME

Protein_____

Fat_____

Veggies_____

Low GI Carb_____

DINNERTIME

Protein_____

Fat_____

Veggies_____

Low GI Carb_____

WATER

☐ ☐ ☐ ☐
☐ ☐ ☐ ☐

EXERCISE

Cardio_____

Strength_____

HOW DO YOU FEEL?

_____
_____
_____
_____
_____
_____
_____
_____
_____
_____
_____
_____
_____
_____

 AFFIRMATION: I love my life. I am so blessed.

Daily Journal

DAY 76

FOOD

BREAKFAST TIME

Protein_____

Fat_____

Veggies_____

Low GI Carb_____

SNACK TIME

Protein_____

Fat_____

Veggies_____

Low GI Carb_____

LUNCH TIME

Protein_____

Fat_____

Veggies_____

Low GI Carb_____

SNACK TIME

Protein_____

Fat_____

Veggies_____

Low GI Carb_____

DINNERTIME

Protein_____

Fat_____

Veggies_____

Low GI Carb_____

WATER

☐ ☐ ☐ ☐
☐ ☐ ☐ ☐

EXERCISE

Cardio_____

Strength_____

HOW DO YOU FEEL?

_____
_____
_____
_____
_____
_____
_____
_____
_____
_____
_____
_____
_____
_____
_____
_____
_____

QUOTE: A dictionary is the only place that success comes before work. Hard work is the price we must pay for success. I think you can accomplish anything if you are willing to pay the price.

~VINCE LOMBARDI

Daily Journal

DAY 77

FOOD

BREAKFAST TIME

Protein_____

Fat_____

Veggies_____

Low GI Carb_____

SNACK TIME

Protein_____

Fat_____

Veggies_____

Low GI Carb_____

LUNCH TIME

Protein_____

Fat_____

Veggies_____

Low GI Carb_____

SNACK TIME

Protein_____

Fat_____

Veggies_____

Low GI Carb_____

DINNERTIME

Protein_____

Fat_____

Veggies_____

Low GI Carb_____

WATER

☐ ☐ ☐ ☐
☐ ☐ ☐ ☐

EXERCISE

Cardio_____

Strength_____

HOW DO YOU FEEL?

_____

_____

_____

_____

_____

_____

_____

_____

_____

_____

_____

_____

_____

_____

_____

_____

 HEALTH TIP: If you are looking to get rid of belly fat, ab work is good, but not the solution. Belly fat is not the result of weak abs; it's too much body fat. The solution is keeping your eating on the right track and exercising the whole body!

Daily Journal

DAY 78

FOOD

BREAKFAST TIME

Protein_____

Fat_____

Veggies_____

Low GI Carb_____

SNACK TIME

Protein_____

Fat_____

Veggies_____

Low GI Carb_____

LUNCH TIME

Protein_____

Fat_____

Veggies_____

Low GI Carb_____

SNACK TIME

Protein_____

Fat_____

Veggies_____

Low GI Carb_____

DINNERTIME

Protein_____

Fat_____

Veggies_____

Low GI Carb_____

WATER

☐ ☐ ☐ ☐
☐ ☐ ☐ ☐

EXERCISE

Cardio_____

Strength_____

HOW DO YOU FEEL?

_____

_____

_____

_____

_____

_____

_____

_____

_____

_____

_____

_____

_____

_____

_____

QUOTE: How does a project get to be a year behind? One day at a time.

~FRED BROOKS

Daily Journal

DAY 79

FOOD

BREAKFAST TIME

Protein_____

Fat_____

Veggies_____

Low GI Carb_____

SNACK TIME

Protein_____

Fat_____

Veggies_____

Low GI Carb_____

LUNCH TIME

Protein_____

Fat_____

Veggies_____

Low GI Carb_____

SNACK TIME

Protein_____

Fat_____

Veggies_____

Low GI Carb_____

DINNERTIME

Protein_____

Fat_____

Veggies_____

Low GI Carb_____

WATER

☐ ☐ ☐ ☐
☐ ☐ ☐ ☐

EXERCISE

Cardio_____

Strength_____

HOW DO YOU FEEL?

_____
_____
_____
_____
_____
_____
_____
_____
_____
_____
_____
_____
_____

AFFIRMATION: I seek progress, not perfection.

Daily Journal

DAY 80

FOOD

BREAKFAST TIME

Protein_____

Fat_____

Veggies_____

Low GI Carb_____

SNACK TIME

Protein_____

Fat_____

Veggies_____

Low GI Carb_____

LUNCH TIME

Protein_____

Fat_____

Veggies_____

Low GI Carb_____

SNACK TIME

Protein_____

Fat_____

Veggies_____

Low GI Carb_____

DINNERTIME

Protein_____

Fat_____

Veggies_____

Low GI Carb_____

WATER

☐ ☐ ☐ ☐
☐ ☐ ☐ ☐

EXERCISE

Cardio_____

Strength_____

HOW DO YOU FEEL?

_____
_____
_____
_____
_____
_____
_____
_____
_____
_____
_____
_____
_____
_____
_____
_____

HEALTH TIP: If you are going to have brown rice, make sure you steam it. Boiling it can make it higher glycemic and put you in fat storage mode.

Daily Journal

DAY 81

FOOD

BREAKFAST TIME

Protein_____

Fat_____

Veggies_____

Low GI Carb_____

SNACK TIME

Protein_____

Fat_____

Veggies_____

Low GI Carb_____

LUNCH TIME

Protein_____

Fat_____

Veggies_____

Low GI Carb_____

SNACK TIME

Protein_____

Fat_____

Veggies_____

Low GI Carb_____

DINNERTIME

Protein_____

Fat_____

Veggies_____

Low GI Carb_____

WATER

☐ ☐ ☐ ☐
☐ ☐ ☐ ☐

EXERCISE

Cardio_____

Strength_____

HOW DO YOU FEEL?

_____
_____
_____
_____
_____
_____
_____
_____
_____
_____
_____
_____
_____
_____
_____

QUOTE: I don't wait for moods. You accomplish nothing if you do that. Your mind must know it has got to get down to work.

~PEARL S. BUCK

Daily Journal

DAY 82

FOOD

BREAKFAST TIME

Protein_____

Fat_____

Veggies_____

Low GI Carb_____

SNACK TIME

Protein_____

Fat_____

Veggies_____

Low GI Carb_____

LUNCH TIME

Protein_____

Fat_____

Veggies_____

Low GI Carb_____

SNACK TIME

Protein_____

Fat_____

Veggies_____

Low GI Carb_____

DINNERTIME

Protein_____

Fat_____

Veggies_____

Low GI Carb_____

WATER

☐ ☐ ☐ ☐
☐ ☐ ☐ ☐

EXERCISE

Cardio_____

Strength_____

HOW DO YOU FEEL?

_____
_____
_____
_____
_____
_____
_____
_____
_____
_____
_____
_____
_____
_____
_____

 AFFIRMATION: I create new positive habits daily.

Daily Journal

DAY 83

FOOD

BREAKFAST TIME

Protein_____

Fat_____

Veggies_____

Low GI Carb_____

SNACK TIME

Protein_____

Fat_____

Veggies_____

Low GI Carb_____

LUNCH TIME

Protein_____

Fat_____

Veggies_____

Low GI Carb_____

SNACK TIME

Protein_____

Fat_____

Veggies_____

Low GI Carb_____

DINNERTIME

Protein_____

Fat_____

Veggies_____

Low GI Carb_____

WATER

☐ ☐ ☐ ☐
☐ ☐ ☐ ☐

EXERCISE

Cardio_____

Strength_____

HOW DO YOU FEEL?

_____

_____

_____

_____

_____

_____

_____

_____

_____

_____

_____

_____

_____

_____

_____

 HEALTH TIP: When buying work-out shoes, now is not the time to shop at the super discount store. Quality shoes are very important for the health of your ankles, knees, hips, and spine!

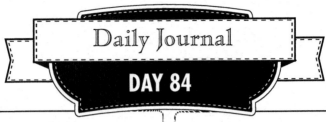

Daily Journal

DAY 84

FOOD

BREAKFAST TIME

Protein_____

Fat_____

Veggies_____

Low GI Carb_____

SNACK TIME

Protein_____

Fat_____

Veggies_____

Low GI Carb_____

LUNCH TIME

Protein_____

Fat_____

Veggies_____

Low GI Carb_____

SNACK TIME

Protein_____

Fat_____

Veggies_____

Low GI Carb_____

DINNERTIME

Protein_____

Fat_____

Veggies_____

Low GI Carb_____

WATER

☐ ☐ ☐ ☐
☐ ☐ ☐ ☐

EXERCISE

Cardio_____

Strength_____

HOW DO YOU FEEL?

_____

_____

_____

_____

_____

_____

_____

_____

_____

_____

_____

_____

_____

_____

_____

_____

TO DO: Measure today!

*Take your "after" picture now. I'd love for you to send them to me…

Week one total inches _____ – week 12 total _____ = total inches lost _____!

PART 4

Recipes

Breakfast
Lunch
Dinner
Sides
Desserts

Breakfast Ziploc Omelets

Good for when you're alone or when all your family is together. The best feature is that no one has to wait for their special omelet. Have the guests write their name on a Quart Size Ziploc <u>Freezer Bag</u> with a permanent marker.

1 Crack 2 eggs into the quart size bag (not more than 2) and shake well.

2 Put out a variety of ingredients such as: cheeses, ham, onions, green peppers, tomatoes, salsa, etc.

3 Everybody adds the prepared ingredients of choice to their bag and shakes the bag to mix them well.

4 Make sure to get the air out of the bag and zip it up.

5 Place the bags into rolling, boiling water for exactly 13 minutes. You can cook 6-8 omelets in a large pot. If you have more omelets, make another pot of boiling water.

6 Cut the bags and the omelet will roll out easily. It's really amazing!

This is a great way to get a low Glycemic break-fast in a hurry. You can make them ahead of time and for a quick breakfast warm it in the microwave.

Breakfast Yogurt

Ingredients:

4-6 oz. Non fat, unsweetened plain yogurt
1 tsp. Ground flaxseed★★
1 tsp. vanilla extract★
½ cup fruit
¼ cup uncooked rolled oats

Directions:

Mix all ingredients and enjoy.

★You can switch vanilla for any flavor you like, maple and almond extracts work nice!

★★You can also switch 1 ½ tablespoon chopped walnuts or other nuts for the flaxseed.

★★★ Greek yogurt has twice the protein, so go for Greek!

Carrot Zucchini Pancakes

I know that sounds crazy but think carrot cake….

Ingredients:

½ cup dry old fashion oatmeal
½ teaspoon ginger, nutmeg, cloves, & baking powder
1 teaspoon cinnamon… or more (I like lots ☺)
1 teaspoon SweetLeaf ® stevia powder (or more)
⅓ cup cottage cheese (or unsweetened applesauce)
3-4 egg whites
Handful of shredded carrots or one sliced carrot
½ peeled zucchini
1 teaspoon vanilla extract and or maple extract (optional)
1 teaspoon coconut oil
Cooking spray

Directions:

Blend all dry ingredients together, in a blender. Then add the rest. Blend until smooth and pour onto a hot griddle or skillet coated with cooking spray. Cook until bubbles pop on the top or when the bottom turns golden brown. No need to top with syrup when you add enough SweetLeaf ® stevia and maple extract.

It doesn't get much easier than that, and you have a healthy carb, protein, fat and a veggie serving.

Quick and Easy Morning Oatmeal

Ingredients:

½ cup dry Old Fashioned Oats
Tsp vanilla or maple extract
10 drops of toffee flavored stevia or ¼ tsp stevia powder
3 egg whites or one whole egg
Enough water to make it soupy

Directions:

Mix all ingredients well and microwave about a 1 ½ minutes. Stir again and cook another 30 seconds to a minute or until it's cooked.

I have this one almost daily so to mix it up a bit I switch the flavored stevia drops for sugar free blueberry syrup and a small handful of frozen blueberries… it's like a fluffy, moist, blueberry muffin without all the fat, calories and processed flour!

One carb and one protein. It's actually a little short on protein unless you use the 3 egg whites version. This will also count as your fat if you include the egg yolk. You decide. ☺

You can always go with egg whites and add walnuts as your fat.

Baked French Toast

4 servings

8 slices of low glycemic bread (I use Ezekiel)
5 egg whites +3 whole eggs
Tsp or 2 of vanilla extract, maple is good here too!
Tsp or so of cinnamon
Tsp of stevia
½ cup milk (I use coconut milk, better flavor and better for you)
Tsp coconut oil, melted
½ cup blueberries (optional)
Cooking spray

Directions:

Preheat oven to 350 degrees. Spray 10x10 cooking dish with cooking spray and place bread slices in the baking dish. You may need to cut the bread to fit in flat. Mix all the other ingredients except blueberries in a bowl and mix well. Top bread slices and top with berries. Bake for about 40 minutes. I find you don't need much syrup, if any ,but of course sugar free is your best bet.. I like to add sugar free blueberry syrup, this is such a yummy treat!

A little carby but pre workout this is a great breakfast..

Eat the Good Fat First

Choosing healthy-fat starters may help you eat less, lose weight.

Eating a small amount of healthy unsaturated fat -- think olive oil, nuts, avocado, and fish -- before a meal triggers a chain reaction in your digestive system that slows the rate at which your stomach empties, which means you feel fuller faster. It also helps keep your blood sugar levels from spiking after your meal and makes it easier for your body to absorb fat-soluble nutrients, such as vitamins A, D, E, and K, as well as lycopene and lutein.

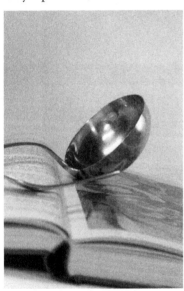

It doesn't take much: Just 70 calories worth will do the trick. That's about ½ tablespoon of olive oil, 6 walnuts, 10 almonds, ¼ of a medium avocado, or 2 ounces of smoked salmon. Just remember, 1 fat choice per meal.

So ditch the chips and instead try some of these delicious **healthy-fat appetizers.**

Spicy Almonds

Makes 2 cups
Serving size: 12 almonds
Calories per serving: 89

Ingredients:

2 tablespoons olive oil
2 cups dry-roasted, unsalted almonds
1 tablespoon Worcestershire sauce
1 tablespoon Splenda ® brown sugar blend
2 teaspoons chili powder
1 teaspoon salt
½ teaspoon cayenne pepper

Directions:

1 Heat the olive oil in a large skillet until hot but not smoking, then add the almonds and stir to combine.

2 Add the Worcestershire sauce, sugar, chili powder, and salt and stir until the almonds are evenly coated.

3 Remove from heat and spread the almonds in an even layer on a baking sheet.

4 Sprinkle them evenly with cayenne pepper and allow to cool.!

Savory Olive Tapenade

Makes 10 servings
Serving size: 2 tablespoons
Calories per serving: 74

Ingredients:

1 teaspoon capers
¾ cup green olives, pitted
¾ cup black olives, pitted
2 cloves garlic, minced
¼ cup olive oil
1 teaspoon lemon juice
2 tablespoons fresh basil, chopped
Pepper, to taste

Directions:

1   Combine all the ingredients in a food processor and pulse until the olives are finely chopped.

2   Serve with baked whole-wheat pita chips or toasted low glycemic bread.

Zesty Pesto Spread

Makes 14 servings
Serving size: 2 tablespoons
Calories per serving: 70

Ingredients:

1 ½ cups fresh spinach leaves
½ cup fresh basil
2 cloves garlic
⅓ cup olive oil
⅓ cup walnuts
2 tablespoons grated Parmesan cheese
Pepper, to taste

Directions:

1   Combine all the ingredients, except the olive oil, in a
    food processor until the mixture is finely chopped.

2   Then, with the food processor running, slowly pour in
    the olive oil until it's all incorporated.

3   Spread onto whole-wheat pita, or even better, sliced
    cucumbers.

★this covers your fat serving

Apple Cheddar Melts on Pita Toast

A nice crisp apple is essential for this snack, so that it won't turn mushy in the oven. Granny Smith or Empire apples are a good choice.

Makes 4 snacks.

Calories: 91, GI: low, Carbs: 14 grams, Protein: 4 grams, Fat: 3 grams. You can lower the fat by using low fat or fat free cheese.

Ingredients:

1 large whole wheat pita bread
4 slices apple
4 slices non-fat cheddar cheese, cut to fit the apple

Directions:

1   Preheat broiler to 400°. Toast one side of the pita. Cut in quarters.

2   Stack the apple slices and cheese slices on each pita. Place back under the broiler until cheese melts.

Ratatouille for Six

Ingredients:

2 tablespoon oil, olive
1 onion, thinly sliced
2 clove(s) garlic, minced
1 eggplant, peeled and diced
2 zucchini, thinly sliced
¾ cup(s) pepper(s), green, bell, diced
2 tomato, chopped
2 tablespoon basil, fresh
¼ teaspoon pepper, black ground
1 tablespoon capers, drained (optional)★

Directions:

1   Heat the oil in a large nonstick skillet. Add the onion and garlic; stir-fry over medium-high heat about 2 minutes.

2   Add the eggplant and stir-fry about 2 minutes. Add the zucchini, green pepper, and tomatoes; stir-fry 3 minutes more.

3   Add the basil, salt, and pepper. Cover and simmer 30 minutes over low heat.

4   Uncover, stir gently, and simmer 10 minutes more. Add the drained capers. Serve hot or chilled.

★ *I love capers, but for this one I'd leave them out. Serve with Chicken breast and whole wheat pasta or quinoa and you have a low Glycemic "fat burning" meal!*

Mini Greek Meatballs

Makes about 24 small meatballs, recipe adapted slightly from "The South Beach Diet Quick and Easy Cookbook."

Ingredients:

1 pound lean ground beef or turkey (use ground beef with less than 10% fat)

½ small onion, minced

½ cup very finely crumbled low fat feta cheese (measure after crumbling finely with a fork) use fat free for weight loss

2 cloves garlic, minced (I used 2 tsp. minced garlic from a jar)

1 large egg or 2 egg whites to lower fat and calories

1 T extra virgin olive oil, plus more for baking dish

1 T dried Greek oregano

4 tsp. red wine vinegar

¼ tsp. salt (optional, I used a tiny bit of Vege-Sal)

¼ tsp. fresh ground black pepper

1 tsp. Greek seasoning, or mint is good too.

Directions:

1   Preheat oven to 400.

2   Use a food processor to chop the onion very finely, then drain if it seems like there is a lot of liquid.

3   Combine all ingredients in a bowl, then use your hands to mix ingredients.

4   Lightly oil a 9 X 13 baking dish. Shape meat into 1 table-spoon size meatballs and place on baking sheet.

5   Bake 20 minutes, after which time you will see some liquid oozing out.

6   Turn meatballs and bake 10 more minutes.

7   Turn again, and bake 5-10 more minutes, until meatballs are well-browned and cooked through.

Awesome Detox Soup

Makes 14 servings
Serving size: 2 tablespoons
Calories per serving: 70

Ingredients:

8-10 cups of water
2cups sliced carrots
1-2 cups green beans
1-2 cups cauliflower
6 or more Tbsp chopped garlic
2 med onions, chopped
2 cups chopped celery
½ chopped green or red pepper
1 cup broccoli, cut in bite size pieces
1 can tomato sauce (low sodium)
1 small can tomato paste
2 Tbsp each dried basil and oregano.
Pepper to taste. If you like cayenne, I would encourage you to add
    that as well.
Handful of fresh chopped spinach
2 cups cabbage

Directions:

1   Combine water, carrots, green beans and cauliflower in
    a large pot. Bring to a boil, and simmer, about 5 minutes.

2   Meanwhile, in a large non-stick pan, sprayed with cooking spray, sauté garlic, onions, and celery until onions become transparent about 5 minutes.

3   Then, to large pot add peppers, broccoli, tomato sauce, tomato paste, basil, oregano and pepper.

4   Simmer another 5 minutes, then add fry pan mixture to pot.

5   Finally add a handful of fresh chopped spinach and 2 cups cabbage.

6   Simmer for another 5 minutes or so until veggies are soft but not mushy.

This is a really good soup and will help you get your detoxing started without the feeling of being deprived at all. Your family will enjoy it as well. Feel free to add any other of your favorite veggies (especially green ones) that you like, just avoid corn, potatoes, rice, beans, pasta, for this week, but if you really like the soup, and I think you will, when you make the soup again, add your proteins or carbs.

Lentil Soup

I like to use lots of carrots, celery in this recipe but if you are not fond of them you can reduce the amounts or lose the carrots and celery and instead throw in some spinach. Experiment on your own with different vegetables, the possibilities are endless, and remember, the more veggies the better!

Makes 8-10 servings.

Ingredients:

2 tbsp olive oil
1 medium onion, chopped
3 carrots, peeled and chopped
3 ribs of celery, chopped
2 cloves garlic, minced
2 cups lentils (about 1 lb)
3 cups water
3 cups chicken broth, reduced fat
28 oz can of diced tomatoes, seasoned
2 large fresh springs of thyme
1 bay leaf
Grated parmesan cheese

Directions:

1 Heat olive oil in a large Dutch oven over medium heat.

2 Add the onion, carrots, celery and garlic and sauté for 10-12 minutes or until tender.

3 Add the lentils, water, chicken broth, diced tomatoes, potatoes, fresh thyme and bay leaf and bring to a boil.

4 Reduce the heat and simmer uncovered for 1 hour or until the lentils are tender.

5 Serve in a bowl and top with grated parmesan cheese.

Similar recipes can be made with green split peas with the elimination of the diced tomatoes. If you don't have fresh thyme on hand, use ½ teaspoon of dried thyme. Also, if the vegetables and lentils aren't soft enough and the liquid is mostly gone add some more chicken broth.

Spicy Yogurt Chicken

Plain yogurt is a magical ingredient in a marinade. It tenderizes chicken while keeping it moist and succulent. Add a little sweetener, something tart and warm spices--and you have a dynamite dish.

4 servings, 2 drumsticks each
Active Time: 15 minutes
Total Time: 1 hour 10 minutes (including ½ hour marinating time)

Ingredients:

2 tablespoons hot water
2 pinches saffron threads, (½ teaspoon)
½ cup nonfat or low-fat plain yogurt
1 onion, very finely chopped
3 cloves garlic, very finely chopped
2 tablespoons harissa, or 2 teaspoons hot sauce or ½ teaspoon cayenne pepper
2 tablespoons lemon juice
1 tablespoon agave syrup
1 tablespoon extra-virgin olive oil
½ teaspoon salt
½ teaspoon ground cumin
¼ teaspoon ground cinnamon
8 chicken drumsticks, skin removed

1 Place hot water in a small bowl and crumble saffron threads over it. Steep for 5 minutes. Combine yogurt, onion, garlic, harissa (or hot sauce or cayenne), lemon juice, honey, oil, salt, cumin and cinnamon in a shallow dish. Stir in the saffron water. Add drumsticks and coat well. Cover with plastic wrap and marinate in the refrigerator for at least 30 minutes or up to 12 hours.

2 Meanwhile, preheat oven to 450°F. Line a baking sheet with foil and set an oiled rack on top. Place the drumsticks on the rack and bake until the chicken is golden brown on the outside and no longer pink in the center, about 30 minutes.

Nutrition

Per serving: 241 calories; 9 g fat (2 g sat, 4 g mono); 82 mg cholesterol; 13 g carbohydrates; 27 g protein; 1 g fiber; 484 mg sodium; 300 mg potassium.

1 Carbohydrate Serving

Exchanges: 3 lean meat, ½ fat

Pinto Bean Salad

Makes 4 carb servings

Ingredients:

1 can pinto beans, rinse and drain very well
4-5 tsp. white balsamic vinegar or champagne vinegar
1 avocado, diced into pieces ½ inch square
2 tsp. fresh lime juice
1 cup chopped tomatoes (cherry tomatoes cut in half would be
    great too, but I had medium tomatoes which I cut in eighths)
½ cup finely chopped red onion
½ cup finely chopped cilantro
1-2 T olive oil, or a bit more
fresh ground black pepper and sea salt to taste

Directions:

1   Pour beans into a colander placed in the sink and rinse
    well until no more foam appears.

2   Let beans drain well for at least 15 minutes.

3   Then blot beans dry with paper towel, place in plastic
    bowl, and toss with white balsamic vinegar.

4   Let beans marinate in the vinegar while you prep other
    ingredients

5 Cut avocado into ½ inch pieces and place in small bowl. Toss with lime juice.

6 Chop tomatoes, or if using cherry tomatoes, cut in half.

7 Chop red onion and cilantro. (I like to chop with a chef's knife, but you could use a mini-chopper or food processor for this.)

8 Mix onions and cilantro into marinating beans. Then use a large spoon to gently fold in avocado and tomato.

9 Drizzle olive oil over salad and season to taste with fresh ground black pepper and sea salt, and gently toss again.

10 Serve immediately, at room temperature

> *Variations: I think other varieties of beans would also be tasty in this combination.*

Chicken with Apples and Leeks

Ingredients:

4 boneless, skinless chicken breast halves (1-1 ¼ pounds), trimmed
3 teaspoons extra-virgin olive oil, divided
¼ teaspoon salt
Freshly ground pepper to taste
2 large leeks, white parts only, washed and cut into julienne strips (2 cups)
2 large cloves garlic, minced
¼ to ½ teaspoon Sweetleaf® stevia
2 teaspoons minced fresh rosemary, or ½ teaspoon dried
¼ cup cider vinegar
2 firm tart apples, such as York or Granny Smith, peeled, cored and thinly sliced
1 cup reduced-sodium chicken broth

Directions:

1 Place chicken breasts between 2 sheets of plastic wrap. Use a rolling pin or a small heavy pot to pound them to a thickness of ½ inch.

2 Heat 1 ½ teaspoons oil in a large nonstick skillet over medium-high heat. Season the chicken breasts with salt and pepper and add to the pan. Cook until browned on both sides, 4 to 5 minutes per side. Transfer to a plate and keep warm.

3 Reduce the heat to low. Add the remaining 1 ½ teaspoons oil and leeks. Cook, stirring, until the leeks are soft, about 5 minutes. Add garlic, sugar and rosemary and cook until fragrant, about 2 minutes more. Increase the heat to medium-high, stir in vinegar and cook until most of the liquid has evaporated.

4 Add apples and broth and cook, stirring once or twice, until the apples are tender, about 3 minutes. Reduce the heat to low and return the chicken and any juices to the pan. Simmer gently until the chicken is heated through. Serve immediately.

Nutrition:

Per serving: 235 calories; 7 g fat (1 g sat, 4 g mono); 64 mg cholesterol; 19 g carbohydrates; 25 g protein; 2 g fiber; 245 mg sodium; 346 mg potassium.

Nutrition Bonus: Selenium (30% daily value), Vitamin A (16% daily value).

1 Carbohydrate Serving

Chicken and Basil

Serves 4 big eaters or 6 medium eaters
Preparation Time 20 - 25 minutes

Ingredients:

4 chicken breasts or 8 chicken thigh fillets
1 Spanish (brown) onion, finely chopped
4 cloves garlic, finely chopped
2 stems of fresh basil leaves, finely chopped or 6 teaspoons basil
    paste or Pesto sauce
A little coconut oil or virgin olive oil is good, but any will do
A selection of vegetables, such as, spinach, chard, broccoli, zuc-
    chini, fresh green french or runner beans,   mushrooms,
    sweet green peppers and Chinese cabbage. Chop these into
    bite size pieces. You can pretty much eat as much of these as
    your family can stand
1 small sweet potato cut into ½ inch of 1cm slices - 4 oz or 125
    gram per serve
1 can Italian tomatoes (no added sugar)

Directions:

1   Gently brown the chicken for 5 to 10 minutes in a frying
    pan with a little oil. Season with salt and black pepper.
    Don't cook all the way through. Remove from the fry-
    ing pan and put to one side.

2   In the same pan, fry the onion and garlic gently, until
    golden brown. Add the basil leaves and canned tomatoes

and put the chicken back into the frying pan. Simmer until the chicken is cooked, about 10- 15 mins. Cut through a piece of chicken to check if it is done.

3   In a separate frying pan, add a little coconut oil, a clove of chopped garlic and the vegetables (not the sweet potato) and fry gently until just tender.(If you prefer a milder garlic flavor, then brown the garlic before adding vegetables.)

4   Add salt and pepper to taste.

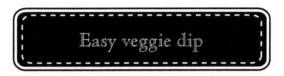

Easy veggie dip

Ingredients:

1 cup nonfat plain yogurt (Greek is best for higher protein) but any will do
1 cup low/non fat feta cheese
1 packet of Ranch salad dressing mix

Directions:

1 Mix all ingredients together and viola, instant veggie dip… enjoy!

**You can add a couple of tablespoons of milk to thin it out for a salad dressing!

Holiday Cranberry Sauce

Ingredients:

12 oz bag of fresh cranberries
1 cup of orange juice
1 ½ to 2 tablespoons SweetLeaf ® stevia powder
1 teaspoon of orange extract
Zest of ½ an orange

Directions:

1 Combine all the ingredients until the cranberries start to pop. Sauce will thicken as it cools... All that yummy flavor without all the sugar!

Refreshing Mango Salsa

Top this cool salsa on your hot grilled chicken breast for an awesome burst of flavor at your next bbq. This will beat out traditional, sugar infested, bbq sauce every time!

Ingredients:

2 mangos
1 avocado
½ cup finely chopped cucumber red onion, & tomato
¼ cup finely chopped red bell pepper, cilantro (I add extra cilantro and)
2 tbls lime juice (or more if you're like me)
1 tbls olive oil and red wine vinegar
Salt and pepper to taste

Directions:

1   Mix and chill. Bring to the next bbq you are invited to and you now not only have a better choice than the regular bbq sauce, you will be the hit of the party!!

Consider this a carb and a fat. All you need now is a nice protein like salmon or chicken and veggies.

Salmon and Broccoli Stir Fry

Ingredients:

½ to a full pound of broccoli florets
½ pound salmon, skin removed, and cut into bite size pieces. Wild caught is best.
1 tablespoon coconut oil
1 teaspoon sesame oil
1 teaspoon of ginger minced
1 garlic clove chopped
Dash of Pickled ginger chopped
⅛ teaspoon SweetLeaf® stevia

Directions:

1 Steam broccoli in the microwave for about 2 minutes in a covered glass bowl.

2 Toss the broccoli and salmon over medium heat with the coconut and sesame oil, cook stirring 2-3 minutes.

3 Add ginger, pickled ginger, stevia, and garlic... sauté another minute and serve!

Goes nice over a serving of brown rice or quinoa as your carb.

Sweet and Sour Chicken Recipe

Ingredients:

1 pound of boneless and skinless chicken thighs or breasts, cut into 1" chunks

1 egg white

½ teaspoon kosher salt (¼ teaspoon table salt) Or Bragg Liquid Aminos

1 10-ounce can pineapple chunks (reserve juice) ¼ cup juice from the canned pineapple

¼ cup white vinegar (no sugar added)

¼ cup ketchup (the kind with no sugar added, Walden Farms make a good one)

½ teaspoon kosher salt (¼ teaspoon table salt)

2 tablespoons Splenda brown sugar blend

¼ cup Walden Farms Sesame Ginger salad dressing

½ tsp SweetLeaf® stevia extract powder (or more)

1 tablespoon + 1 teaspoon coconut oil

1 large carrot, (a handful of shredded carrots works too) and 2 zucchinis cut into bite size pieces

8-10 oz bag of shredded cabbage

box sliced mushrooms

½ onion, cut into small bite size chunks

1 red or yellow bell pepper, cut into 1 inch chunks (or both)

1 teaspoon grated fresh ginger

You can certainly add any of your other favorite veggies, I added snow peas....

If you like spicy, like me, I added a teaspoon or two of chili garlic sauce

1 In a bowl, combine the chicken with the egg white & salt. Stir to coat the chicken evenly. Let it sit for 15 minutes at room temperature or up to overnight in the refrigerator.

2 In the meantime, whisk together the pineapple juice, vinegar, sesame ginger dressing, ketchup, salt, and brown sugar blend, and stevia.

3 Heat a large frying pan or wok over high heat until a bead of water instantly sizzles and evaporates. Pour in the 1 tablespoon of coconut oil and swirl to coat. It's important that the pan is very hot. Add the chicken and spread the chicken out in one layer. Let the chicken fry, untouched for 1 minute, until the bottoms are browned. Flip and fry the other side the same for 1 minute. The chicken should still be pinkish in the middle. Dish out the chicken onto a clean plate, leaving as much oil in the pan as possible.

4 Turn the heat to medium and add the remaining 1 teaspoon of coconut oil. Let the oil heat up and then add the bell pepper chunks, zucchini, mushrooms, cabbage, (and any other veggies) and ginger. Fry for 1 minute. Add the pineapple chunks and the sweet and sour sauce. Turn the heat to high and when the sauce is simmering, add the chicken pieces back in. Let simmer for 1-2

minutes, until the chicken is cooked through. Timing depends on how thick you've cut your chicken. The best way to tell if the chicken is done is to take a piece out and cut into it. If it's pink, add another minute to the cooking. Serves 4.

This is a complete meal! Remember, 1 protein, 1 carb, 1 fat, and lots of veggies per meal….no need to add any rice… You have your protein in the chicken, carb is your pineapple, your fat is your coconut oil and lots of veggies…

And this one is really good! ☺ Eating healthy doesn't have to taste like cardboard!!

*For more on eating healthy and weight loss
made easy visit www.TamiLindahl.com*

Creamy Cauliflower Purée

Vegan, gluten free

A terrific substitute for heavy, high glycemic, butter-laden potatoes, this light take on mashed spuds serves up fewer than half the calories but with all of the flavor. Make these your new holiday tradition and don't tell—your guests may not even realize they aren't eating potatoes.

Ingredients:

1 large head cauliflower, cut into 1- to 2-inch florets (5–6 cups)
2–4 cloves garlic, peeled
2 cups low-sodium vegetable broth or water
1 tsp gray sea salt, plus more when puréeing
¼ cup olive oil
¼ tsp freshly ground pepper
1 heaping tbsp fresh herbs, to garnish

Directions:

1   In large sauce pot or steamer, place cauliflower, garlic, broth or water and sea salt. Cover and bring to boil, then reduce heat and simmer 10–15 minutes or until tender. Stir occasionally to ensure even cooking. Drain, reserving cooking liquid.

2   Puree in two batches in food processor until smooth, scraping down sides as needed. With motor running, add ¼ cup cooking liquid, half the olive oil, pepper and

pinch of sea salt to each batch. Adjust seasoning to taste. Transfer to serving dish, top with herbs and serve hot. Can be made ahead and kept warm or reheated on low. Serves six.

Note: I added a couple of dollops of plain non fat yogurt and a splash of butter extract and it was really good! You can add any seasonings you would normally add to mashed potatoes... these are really good.

Black Bean Brownies

This sounds pretty ridiculous, but you will be absolutely amazed at how good they are!!

Makes 16 brownies (approx 1 ½ per serving)

Ingredients:

2 cups cooked black beans drained(you can substitute with 1 can of black beans)
4 eggs or 6-7 egg whites (to reduce fat)
2 tbsp coconut oil
1 tbsp vanilla
sugar substitute – equivalent to 1 cup (I used Splenda for Baking)
3 tbsp cocoa powder (I used Hershey's)
¼ tsp salt
½ tsp baking powder
walnuts/pecan chopped (optional)
non stick cooking spray

Directions:

1   Heat the oven to 350 degrees F. Lightly spray an 8 x 8 baking pan with non stick cooking spray.

2   In a blender or food processor, combine the black beans, eggs, oil, vanilla, sugar substitute, cocoa powder, baking powder, and salt. Process until smooth.

3   Scrape the batter into the baking pan and sprinkle the nuts on top. Bake for 25 to 30 minutes in the preheated

oven, until a toothpick inserted in the center comes out clean.

4 Cut into 16 squares.

Nutrition per Brownie: 34 Calories, 2g Fat, 0.4g Sat, 1g Protein, 2g Carbs, 1g Fiber, 66mg Sodium

Resources

For Fitness tips, recipes and weight loss coaching:
www.TamiLindahl.com

Fitness/dance videos:
www.Jillina.com

Nutritional information on most foods:
www.nutritiondata.com

Inspirational T-shirts and products:
www.SheriBabyTshirts.com

Glycemic index:
www.glycemicidex.com

Healing Jewelry:
www.charityclarityjewelry.com

Fitness Equipment:
www.Fitterbodiesinc.com

Sugar free chocolate for weight loss
http://tinyurl.com/bw9thsh

CPSIA information can be obtained
at www.ICGtesting.com
Printed in the USA
FSOW04n2207050515
6870FS